THYMUS
ACTIVATION HEALING

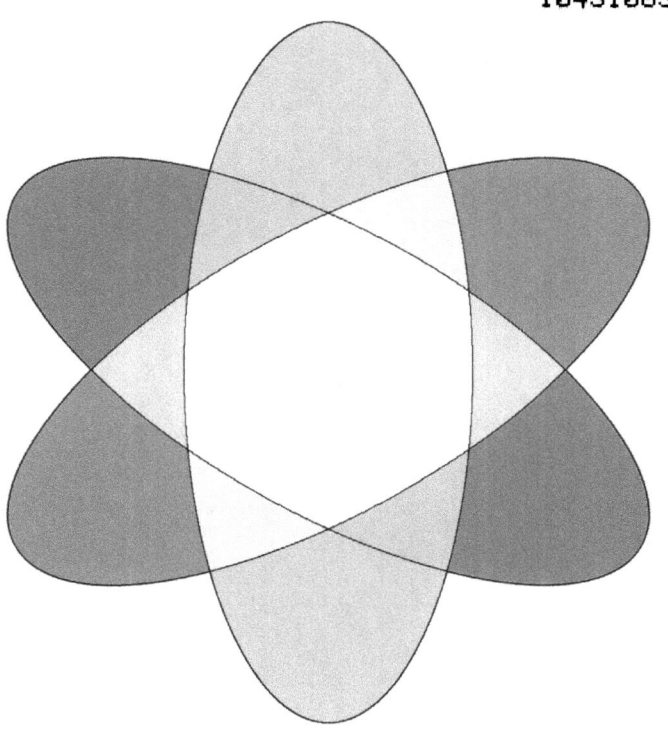

MR.
TAKASHI 2BAKI

Thymus activation healing English only version 1.0 revision 2

Mr. Takashi 2baki

INTRODUCTION

The method of thymus activation healing is introduced at the end of the book.

If you want to try healing as soon as possible, please go to the end page.

First, I would like to introduce you to love, which is the cornerstone of healing.

Next, I will introduce what happened as a result of continuing the healing.

Next, I will introduce the healing that I have been taught and the healing that I have devised independently.

Next, I will make a hypothesis and introduce information about the thymus from a medical point of view.

In conclusion, I will introduce how to perform thymus activation healing.

By all means, I hope that you will proceed without resistance.

I hope you enjoy this book.

TABLE OF CONTENTS

Introduction	3
Table of contents	5
Love	6
Hermit story	12
Ascension	19
Kagome	23
Awakening experience	32
Relief policy	37
Foreword	70
Main story	71
Literature list	84
Service	86
Hypothesis	96
Thymus	104
At the end	143

LOVE

This is the tested version of love.

What do you think of when you hear the word love? The love of romance, the love of friendship, the love you feel in acts of kindness, and so on. I can imagine that kind of love.

In this, I think that self-love is included if you tell one more true love.

Self-love

It is self-loving love.

Self-love creates spiritual independence.

In other words, loving yourself is nourishing your body. And at the same time, you receive the nourishment of love for your body.

for this body. It has never been so reliable.

Giving love and receiving love, such a cycle sprouts in one individual, and when a loop of love energy is born, this body becomes a state full of joy, and you will be happy from the bottom of your heart.

If you continue to do this on a daily basis, it will become a signpost for your spiritual independence and will lead you to an upward rise.

This is called ascension.

Or we call it an updraft.

And experience true self-love.

When you wake up to true self-love, you will be able to live without depending on others. You can live simply with self-love without receiving love from others.

And, well, that's what happens.

Of course, we receive a lot of love from others and are able to enjoy even more love, so it's like killing two birds with one stone.

Therefore, there is no reason not to obtain this. I think so. By all means, please check it with your own eyes.

About the definition of love

Even if you say love in one word, I think there are various perceptions.

Love in romantic relationships, love in friendship, love in acts of sincerity and kindness.

What we can infer from these things is that love works like a socially proven lubricating oil (lubricant, grease) to enrich human life.

Here, I would like to offer an energetic perspective on this working of love. I would like to proceed with a new definition of the existence that exists in the heart, the center of the chest, the human center core (heart), and the existence that can be inherent in the self.

The purpose of this article is for you to experience the use of the energy of your own being, the being that resides in your heart, and experience the circulation of the energy of love. And I would be happy if you could become an awakener of the energy of love.

Also, if you can handle the energy of love freely, you will be able to reduce anxiety first. Of course, you can't get rid of anxiety completely, but the energy of love will be revitalized, so it's healthier than going to a bad psychiatrist. A healthy effect can be expected.

Also, when the energy of love circulates throughout the body, skin rejuvenation and beauty effects can be expected.

We will be protected by gentle and warm circulating energy, so I think we will be able to declare that we are safe no matter how much confusion the world may have.

Also, when you become able to use the energy of love, you will come to know that there is an energy existence inherent in all things that exist in this world.

When that happens, you will come to be able to treat things naturally and with care, because you will know that there is an existence that is inherent in all things, just like yourself.

And since you will no longer perceive things as mere things, you will be able to love the existence that is inherent in those things. Then, I think that attitudes such as throwing away things poorly or not treating them with care will disappear.

Also, if you come to know that there is an existence inherent in things, I think that you will be less likely to want, steal, or loot other people's things.

It is because we know that there is an existence that is inherent in the object, and we will naturally notice that the existence loves its master (owner), so the feelings of the existence that is inherent in the object will naturally come to us.

I think that people will stop coveting, stealing, and plundering other people's things.

I think that this is not just a thought for things, but a way of thinking that can be applied to people as well. I think it's similar to a situation where you can't get your hands on someone, assuming that you've found someone you like, but that person also likes someone else. Even if you know that your love will never come true, you will probably stop wanting or stealing someone else's lover.

Also, when you learn to think with love, you will be able to perceive things with your heart. Therefore, I know that even the person I hate who is with the person I love is someone who has the potential to be a "precious" being who can use love in the same way as I do. Therefore, I think that envy and jealousy will decrease. To take an extreme example, I think the tragic appearance of killing people just because they hate them will disappear.

I think that there is the true value of love.

Also, when you are ready to use the energy of love, an upward current (ascension) will occur.

From the next chapter, I would like to introduce some of the experiences and tell you how to use the energy of love and friendship.

HERMIT STORY

In the past, I began to see that this might be the reason why the people called hermits were all advocating immortality.

I will write about this in this chapter.

It is said that the meaning of immortality is to never grow old and never die.

But the old hermits are dying. I'm starting to think that what they wanted to say was that they were able to realize a way of life that looked youthful without getting old, and that they were expressing it in words.

As long as we are human, we are bound to die, but I think that the hermits may have devised a way to stay youthful forever by using the latent abilities that humans are endowed with.

As a result, I speculate that he became a being called a hermit who is said to never die.

So they discovered something that they couldn't understand at the level of common sense or modern science, and they were familiar with it. That's what I think. However, although I've seen stories about hermits in books, I've never met a real hermit, so I thought of them as little more than fairy tales.

However, I learned crystal healing from Mr. Robert Simmons, who is famous in the natural stone industry. As the saying goes, if you like what you do, you are good at it. As a result of continuing crystal healing every day, I had an ascension experience. In other words, it means that I experienced the rising air current at a level that I can feel in my body.

As a result, the story of the "invisible system" world has become more realistic. The human body really has a lot of secrets, and it seems that there really is an unknown area that has not been elucidated by science.

In the past, I was also a realist, the type of person who didn't pay much attention to stories about invisible systems. However, when you really experience ascension, you can't ignore it, and you're in the current situation that you want to send it yourself.

This is a real story. I was really surprised.

As for me, once I tasted the ascension experience, I began to ascend every day without fail. As for the method of healing, I have devised a unique method of healing without crystals, and I am still brushing it up by applying it to the method of using the energy of love and friendship.

In the midst of this, from around mid-May to early June 2022, I had the climax of my ascension experience, an awakening experience with fear. This is a very difficult content to convey, but the diametrically opposite phenomenon that is inextricably linked to joy has emerged. This requires extreme caution.

In that experience, I experienced the activation of existence in a place that is difficult to describe in words, slightly above the center of my heart.

From this, I became interested in what this was, and when I looked up all the medical books in the library, it seems that it is what is called the thymus in the medical world. I understood that it was the thymus.

From this experience, it has become clear that the thymus is an organ that matures T cells that control human immune functions. Diseases such as cancer and corona will be advantageous if even the thymus can be activated. You will be able to say that.

From this, if the activation of the thymus occurs, the immune function will go up. And if you can progress to the awakening experience, you will be able to recognize the existence of the thymus with skin sensation. You will be able to activate the thymus by practicing the use of the energy of love and friendship every day. I'm starting to be able to say that.

I'll make a supplement. I described it as being able to perceive the sensation of the thymus. but this has a special meaning.

In the actual process of awakening, my body became too sensitive and I felt like I was transcending gender. As a result, in the process of activating various organs, I sensed a sensation that resembled a "butterfly" in the upper part of my chest (thymus).

In my case, I feel that it can be described as a "hinge", and I also feel that it can be likened to a wing. I think some people perceive it like a bird. Perhaps, I imagine that the way people see and feel will change depending on the person.

Therefore, I think that various ways of expression other than those expressed here will appear in the world in the future. I had such a special feeling.

Of course, I think we need to demonstrate this. However, I am neither a doctor nor a medical practitioner. So I have no idea how to prove it. Also, it will be necessary to verify whether it is an awakening experience that happened only to me or an experience that can happen to anyone. In my experience, it takes three years to experience awakening.

If we try to prove this in the form of verification or clinical trials, how many years will it take until the technology system is established? Whether or not I can prove it in my lifetime is also unknown at this point.

So, now that you are reading this article, you are in luck.

If you read this article and would like to have an ascension experience or an awakening experience, please read the rest of this book carefully. I would like to introduce you to how to use the energy of love and friendship.

Going back to the original story, I imagine that the ancient hermits learned the activation of the thymus through this awakening experience and lived by making the most of this experience. It's just a hypothesis, but I'm imagining that if I had this experience about 500 years ago when medical care was at the level of the past, I might have become like a hermit.

In modern times, the level of medical care has risen too much, and it is changing to an era that is even said to be "an era in which we cannot die." Therefore, we are now in an era where we can solve problems with the power of medicine without becoming a hermit.

However, if you can live long with the natural healing power of human beings, it would be better to use the power of natural healing power. Then I would like to introduce the essence of the main story.

From here, I would like to introduce the experience of the rising air current (ascension) and the relief policy, including the story at the time of the awakening experience.

ASCENSION

The updraft (ascension) experience may look and feel different depending on the person. I would appreciate it if you could treat the contents I will introduce from now on as "one example". Please understand in advance that what I am going to tell you about will not necessarily happen.

I will tell you as my experience story.

In mid-July 2019, I attended a certain seminar. That's where I met Crystal Healing. Since then, I have continued to practice crystal healing on a daily basis.

About three months later, before the first Ascensions began, I would like to share with you what struck me as something that happened. When I was doing crystal healing, I saw an image of a large lotus flower blooming from the base, or rather, from the center between the legs, and the petals opening.

Also, when the first ascending air current (ascension) began, I felt a brilliant light in the center of my heart in my slumber. It was like looking into the center of your heart in a dreamy state.

I recognize that around this time, I was able to clearly recognize the existence inherent in myself, feel the sense of reality with my skin, and face the wonder of the human body.

When I first experienced the rising air currents (ascension) rising into my heart, I was truly astonished.

It's like saying, "What the hell is this?"

Since that experience, stories about invisible systems, ascension, vibrational rise, and dimensional ascension that have been talked about in the streets can happen to anyone, not to specific crazy people. I know it's an event.

Also, when the rising air current (ascension) was approaching the throat above the heart.

I was surprised to hear the sound of "Ah————n", low deep bass, solid midrange sound, faint high-pitched sound, and surround sound as if many voices were chanting together. I still remember that.

Up to this point, I remember that it happened about 3 to 6 months after I started crystal healing.

Also, about half a year after starting crystal healing, I was able to use the energy of love without using crystals. Since then, I have practiced using the energy of love and friendship without crystals.

In terms of period, I practiced crystal healing for half a year, and practiced how to use the energy of love and friendship for about two years and four months. 2 years and 10 months in total.

In the process of continuing the updraft (ascension), at some point, the updraft (ascension) began to occur up to the inside of the skull above the throat.

Two years and ten months later,

The Ascension bestows a ray of hope as it moves further into the skull. However, it can also be a picture of hell for some people. I struggled.

As a result, even though I had been given the saying, "The one who advances without resistance wins," I faced a gender-transcending physical situation that made me unable to resist. Despite the language, I reached the limit of my patience, and for the first time I resisted the phenomenon that occurred in my body.

And then, tormented by chills, fear, and anxiety, he faced a moment when he was prepared to die. I will keep the details secret, but it was truly a picture of hell.

And I'm a man I'm a man I was driven to the point where I started saying a spell, and I just endured it.

And from here, we will rush into the awakening experience.

KAGOME

Kagome, Kagome, Kago no naka no tori wa, itu itu deyaru Yoake no ban ni, turu to kame ga subetta, ushiro no syoumen daare. *This is written in Japanese pronunciation.

If you're Japanese, it's a song that you often played as a play song when you were a child. However, when I read it after going through an ascension experience, I was surprised by the contents of the song, and realized that it was a little different from the impression I had when I was a child. This chapter will tell you about this.

This song seems to have a slightly different word depending on the region. Most of them say the same thing, so I will apply the words introduced at the beginning of this chapter to express them.

Kagome, I definitely took this word as a childhood play song that was blindfolded and surrounded by a large number of people. However, after experiencing the updraft (ascension) and reading it, I realize that it doesn't mean that at all.

Kagome, Kagome, this kagome means basket eyes, basket eyes. Well, it's a picture of a mixture of triangles and inverted triangles, in the shape of a six-pointed star.

So what does "Kago no naka no tori wa" mean? The meaning can be annotated in various ways. The first is Torii. Torii means a gate built at the entrance of a shrine.

From my ascension experience, this is the "hinge" part. In terms of medical terms, it is the thymus that lives slightly above the heart, which is also the center core of humans.

It looks like a bird depending on how you look at it.

I felt like a "butterfly" when I experienced the updraft (ascension). However, depending on how you look at it, it may look like a bird. Even if I express it as a bird, I don't feel any sense of incongruity. Both are flying beings. So the second is a bird.

And then, "itu itu deyaru Yoake no ban ni" This means, perhaps, when? When? Can you show me what it looks like? It's dawn night. I take it as meaning that it expresses the unbearable state of anticipation and confusion.

It was the night before dawn when I first felt the hot, energetic "butterfly" (thymus).

At the climax of the ascension, which leads to an awakening experience, I could clearly feel the heated "butterfly".

And about the meaning of "turu to kame ga subetta," I take this word to mean that the turtle slipped smoothly, not the crane.

To explain it pictorially, I think there is a picture like a tortoise shell inside a six-pointed star that is Kagome, but I would like you to rotate it slightly. Then you can see it.

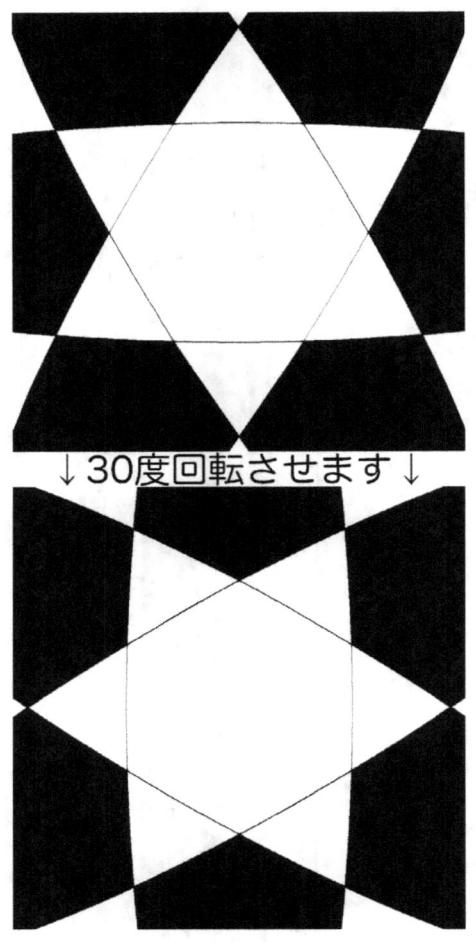

And, "ushiro no syoumen daare" This is a story that can be understood by those who have experienced the ascension experience and the awakening experience, but I think it is quite difficult to understand generally.

If the torii (entrance) of Kagome is expressed as the thymus, then the main hall (worship hall) of Kagome is the top of the head. Well, it's hard to put into words. It can also be expressed as the position of Enma, the position of the crown, or the position of the beans.

From my personal point of view, I see "ushiro no syoumen daare" as the existence that is inherent in oneself.

Description of Kagome

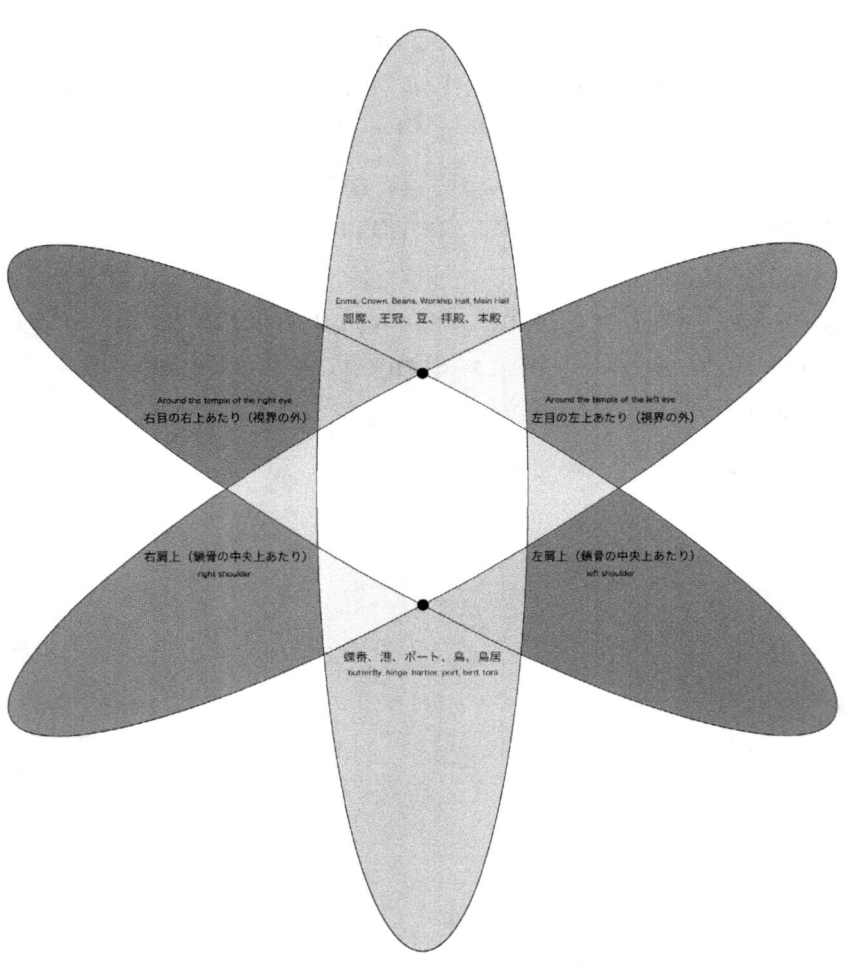

Also, when you hear the word Enma, you may think of something scary.

There is also the influence of stories such as Dragon Ball and Journey to the West, and that is how it is perceived, but for people who have experienced ascension and awakening, Enma looks a little different.

Enma means a beautiful person who is extremely enthusiastic about one thing. I would be happy if the impression of Enma changed even a little.

Also, the crown refers to the circular wide part of the sagittal suture that connects the parietal bones to the parietal bones. It will appear after continuing the ascension experience.

Also, the suffering of hell will appear ahead of continuing the upward current (ascension). Beans will appear at the end of that hellish suffering.

Words cannot explain it at all, so to explain it in medical terms, the suture between the frontal bone in the skull and the left and right parietal bones is called the coronal suture.

The point where the coronal suture and sagittal suture intersect will be referred to as the bean position.

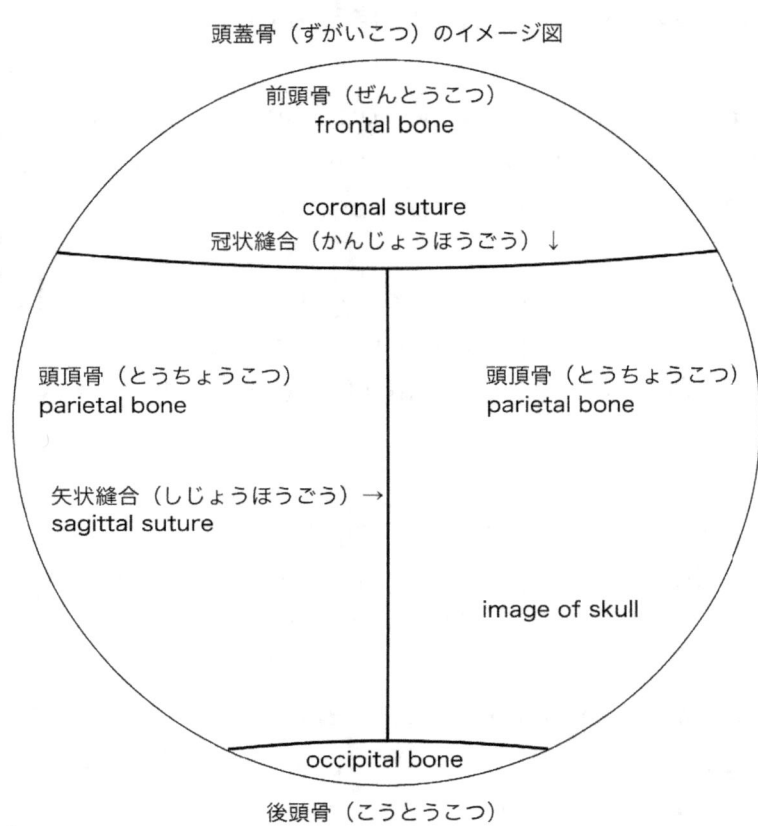

I would appreciate it if you could convey it

However, I am impressed that the old people said well. When I was a child, I was made to sing and play with that song, and I was educated properly.

Moreover, the meaning of play and the meaning of inner exploration are well combined, and it is too wonderful to have two meanings.

It exactly contains the rising air (ascension) itself, and I don't know who thought of it, but it's good.

I thought the person who wrote the song was a genius.

Then, from the next chapter, I will introduce the story of the time when I had a crazy awakening experience after proceeding with the ascension experience.

AWAKENING EXPERIENCE

love and friendship. When you know how to use that energy, the updraft (ascension) will come to happen.

When you can master the ascending air current, it evolves from the ascending air current around the navel to the ascending air current that rises to the chest (heart) and rises to the throat and then to the head. It becomes a pattern that moves to the top of the head, and in the process of moving to the top of the head, it becomes a "super ascension", and it becomes like holding a bean in exchange for hellish suffering. This requires caution and self-recovery.

When this happens, the desire to ascend will disappear. Rather, it struggles desperately to balance the heart and the head (maala). That is the pattern of being showered with cold water.

As a result, I seem to let go of everything, even my imagination. It also begins to obscure all the knowledge it has gained in its inner search.

I am in that state right now.

I'll show you what I'm doing now

The past and the future are all dreams.
Fantasies and delusions are the same as dreams.
Even memories are dreams.
If you notice that, say it out loud right now.
Focus on the visible world.
The visible world is real.
The visible world is the present reality.
So, when you start chasing the invisible world, I want you to say it out loud right now.
Focus on the visible world. And if you do that, your eyes will be bright and there will be no aftereffects.

Now your head starts syncing to the present.

There is something I want you to do next. Try to follow your breathing. You don't have to think about how many seconds to exhale and how many seconds to inhale. I'm exhaling air now. I'm getting air now When you start the live commentary, the head and body synchronized with the present will start to work together. There is a state that a space of the heart is born here.

And, well, when it comes to this state, it makes me feel better. If you find yourself in a state of uncontrollable confusion after mastering Ascension, please read this article. Your mind and body will surely be reset.

I will explain what happened after I wrote this sentence.

As a result of letting go of everything, and even letting go of imagination, perhaps the preparations for the body were complete, and all at once they were in a state of letting go of even the sensations of their bodies.

It's called the secret formula and it's the way everyone goes.

It happened against my will. And I don't even know if I'm breathing or not, I can't even feel my body, it's just there. But here it is. It was only the feeling of saying.

It is a feeling that even thoughts do not exist.

Then, when I thought my head was twitching, the sense of my body returned, I felt shallow breathing, and my thoughts returned.

What is this? ⋯ Ultimately, I search for words that are similar to this experience from my past experience memories, but even if I come up with various words and try to apply them, the moment I apply them, the words has become a sense of lying. I noticed the contradiction of explaining in words. I came to think that naming it would be a lie.

I feel like I'm subconsciously immersed in meditation⋯, Putting it into words would be a lie.

For the time being, just to be sure, I will list only what I thought at that time, with the meaning of not forgetting my original intention.

It's a feeling of peace⋯, Is this what you mean by "nothing"? Is this Samadhi? However, I can't help but see nothingness and samadhi as false words. If you write "nothing", you can conclude that it is not "nothing" because it has the feeling of "it is just here." It seems that the word samadhi means to focus one's mind on one thing and achieve a stable state of mind, but I myself do not feel that my mind is focused on one thing at all. This state of affairs occurs arbitrarily regardless of one's will, so it is probably not samadhi.

Well, what is this, as a result of the analysis, I conclude that this state cannot have a name. It can be described as the ultimate in ecstasy, but you notice that the impression of the words you are conveying has changed. It may be misleading to those who read this sentence for the first time. If you look only at that part, it looks fake. Also, if you analyze whether it is bliss, it seems that it means supreme happiness (satisfaction of the heart)⋯, No, that's not what I mean⋯, As a result, it may be in such a state, but it is not such an impression physically and emotionally⋯

Putting it into words would be a lie. It can be said that it is a state that cannot be expressed in words, but what is it in the end? If you ask me, I can't explain.

I felt that way.

I have some thoughts from those experiences.

"Well, thinking itself was a dream."

If you are interested in the updraft (ascension) after reading this text and want to experience it, please experience how to use the energy of love and friendship.

Whether or not this works for you is up to you. We hope you enjoy it.

RELIEF POLICY

When you begin to enjoy the updraft called the Ascension, you will experience the updraft below the belly button (Ascension), the updraft in the heart (Ascension), the updraft in the throat (Ascension), and the updraft in the skull (Ascension). When that happens, you will begin to experience the joys and sorrows that are the exact opposite of the joys and happiness that you used to have.

The more you do ascension, the more you suffer. You get chills. It will be in a mentally cornered state to quit healing. Well, you start having the kind of symptoms that are medically diagnosed as schizophrenia or depression.

So be careful.

In my case, I just happened to like reading, and the books I read helped me. I would like to introduce the results in my own words.

The state of worrying about the past and the future is called mind wandering.

As a result of experiencing the ascending air currents (ascension) entering into the skull, I was attacked by chills, fear and anxiety, and fell into a mentally cornered state. As a result, I became aware that I was pursuing the invisible world too much, and changed my consciousness to pursue the visible world and started to spend my normal life.

In the meantime, I will write what I noticed.

Up until now, when my memories of the past appeared fragmentary in the form of images, I would remember them forever and ponder what it was like at that time. Such a repetition, a loop, was actually a form of pursuing an invisible world. I've come to realize that. I return to chasing the visible world. After declaring this, I returned and discovered that I had been tormented by this until now. I realized that memories of the past are memorized data, and fantasies inflated with images, in other words, delusions.

If you understand that, for example, if you win the first prize in the lottery, your imagination, in other words, your delusion, is a form of excessive pursuit of things you can't see. I had a realization. Well, this too was nothing more than a vision of the future that I hoped would be like this. It's proof that you're chasing too much of what you can't see. I had a realization.

To be honest, this made me feel better. However, just by changing your consciousness to pursue what you can see, you can change your consciousness considerably. I'm starting to think.

In any case, I think it would be great if I could get into the habit of resetting by saying that once I start pursuing the invisible (the past and the future), I will return to the consciousness of pursuing the visible world.

But just in case you find yourself falling into chills, fears, and insecurities that returning to the pursuit of the visible just can't resolve, here's what you need to know.

It is this.

The secret of the ring finger. relaxation method. It's a way to unwind.

Each of the five fingers on the hand has its own usage and meaning. I will introduce it while quoting it.

Yagyu Shinganryu
■ Talking about the fingers of the hand, there are three streams of muscle fibers in the hand.
The first is the flow of the thumb,
The second is the flow of the index finger and middle finger,
The third is the flow of the ring finger and little finger.
〜The meaning of each finger〜

・ Thumb: strong power, the thumb is the last to rely on. (Use only when you want to convey power)

・ Index finger: power to extend

・ Middle finger: Spinning finger. Rotate around your middle finger. Hands are easier to turn.

・ Ring finger: Only the ring finger has sympathetic and parasympathetic nerves. sensitive. The most sensitive.

・ Little finger: Ability to gather together: When you hold it with your little finger, it will come together.

Quote source
https://www.youtube.com/watch?v=8H6LtISZ8Bw

I'm not a martial artist, so I don't hit people, but I was interested in the meaning of fingers and how to use them. I felt that it could be used for anything, so I started researching on my own. I will introduce what I have learned in it.

If you are assuming that you will hit, such as martial arts, I think it will be a form of holding the little finger and the ring finger.

A form that assumes hitting

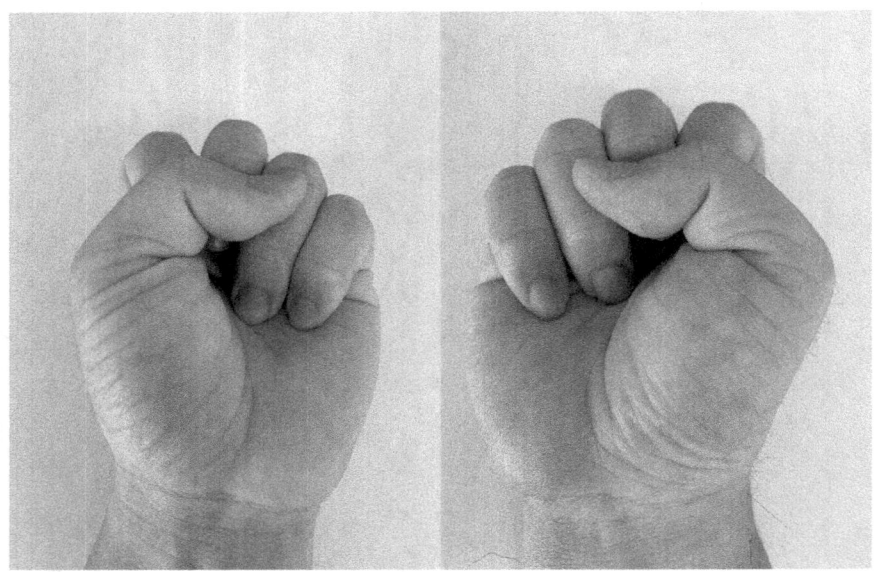

However, with this, the little finger and the ring finger inevitably put a lot of force, so when I tried walking, it became easier, but I felt that the shoulder was a little strained, so I continued to improve it. As a result, I devised a grip method that does not grip. For walking only.

form that does not grip

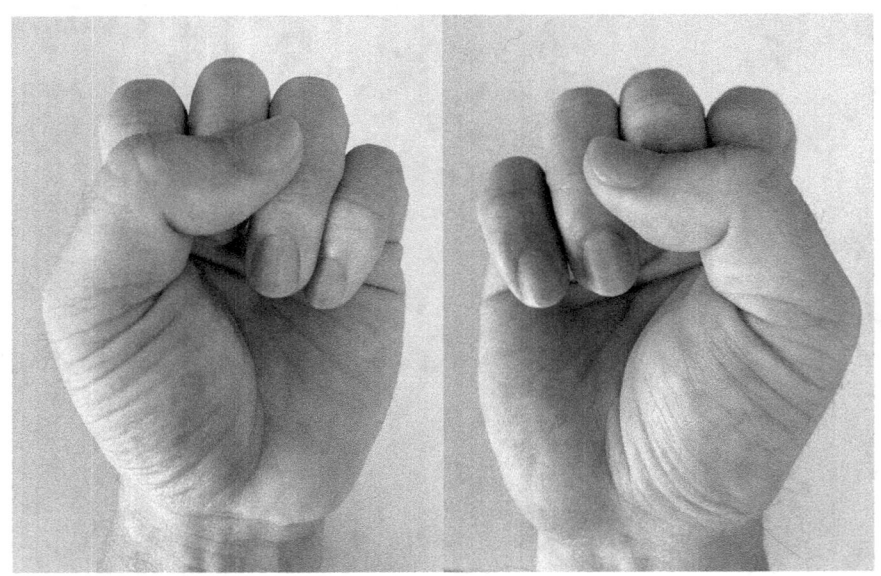

The important thing is to feel the thumb lightly touch the ring finger, and to have an image of lightly attaching it, and not to force it so as not to grip it.

Next, I will introduce how to use the ring finger, which is usually useful for ordinary people. It puts the pad of the thumb on the nail of the ring finger so that it touches lightly. Leave it as it is with no effort. Then, the tension in your shoulders will go away, and you will feel the sensation of stretching all the way down to your toes.

The effect is great.

original form of discovery

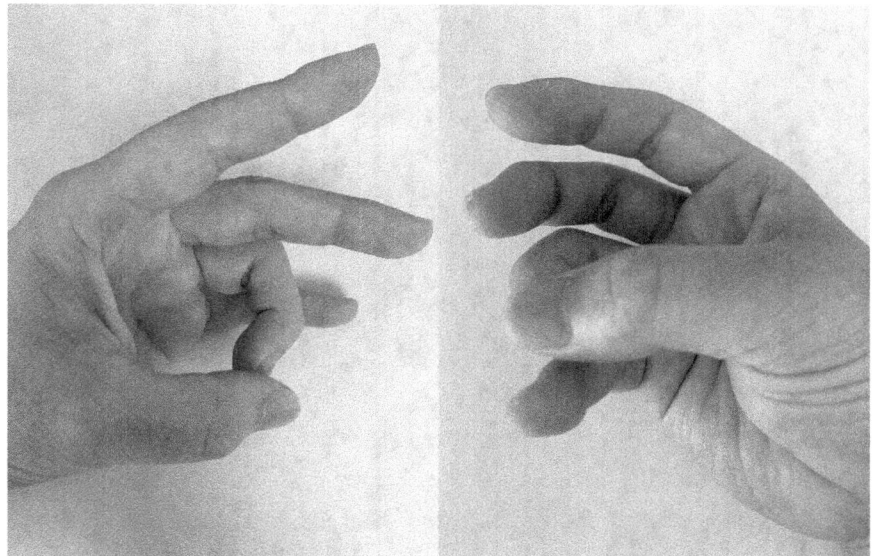

This is what happened when I got used to it. However, the sensation of stretching all the way to your toes will diminish.

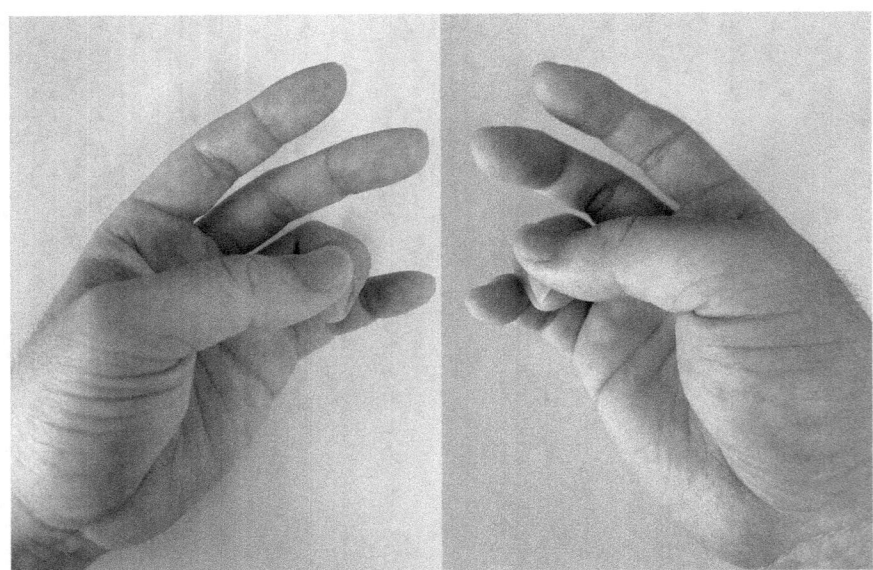

I feel that the opposite phenomenon occurs when I put the pads of my fingers together instead of putting them on my nails. I feel like my hands are tingling, my hands are trembling, and I feel like I'm in a state of excitement. You should be careful.

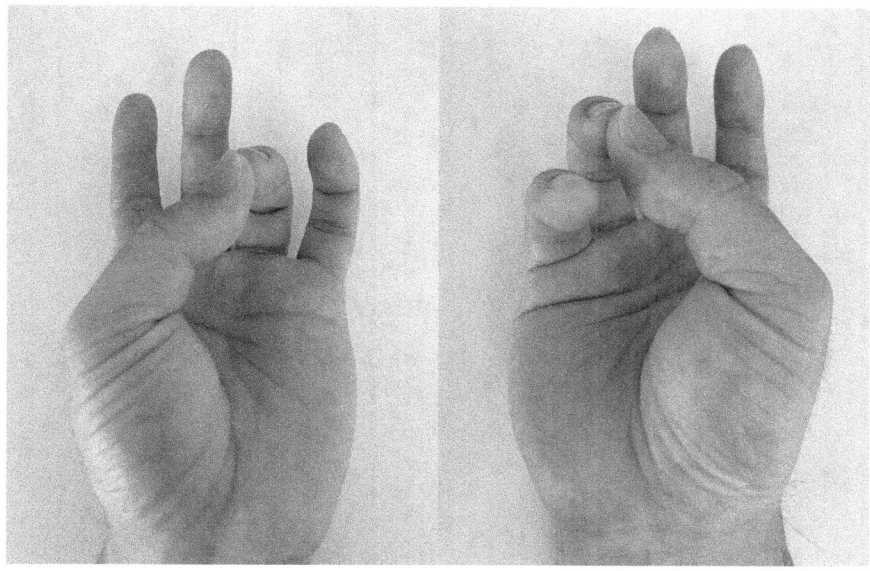

If you put your thumb on the nail and skin of your ring finger, it will naturally become a piece. I felt like my shoulders and neck were being protected.

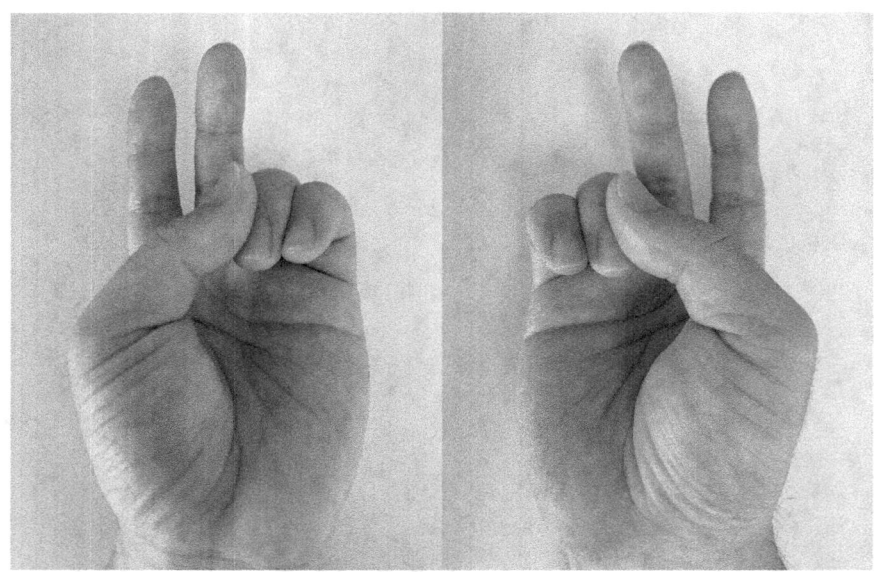

Lightly touch the first joint of the ring finger with the tip of the pad of the thumb to create a state in which the thumb touches the joint of the ring finger. Then, lightly place the pad of your thumb so that it touches the nail of your ring finger. It's a really small difference, but it makes a big difference.

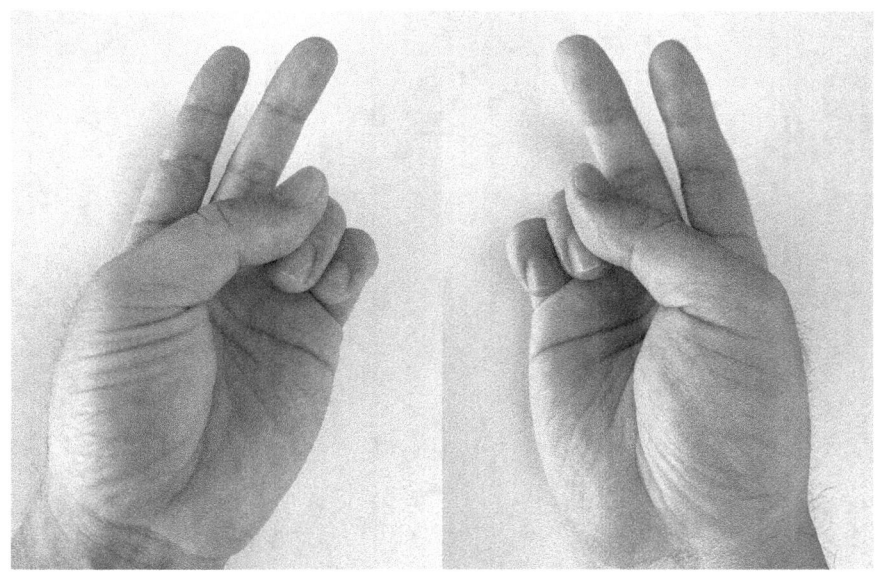

I'm so impressed with this.

When I touched the back of my ring finger with the pad of my thumb, I felt my whole body relax and even my mind became stable. I'm hypothesizing that the parasympathetic nervous system is in a dominant state. Also, perhaps, I hypothesize that the sympathetic nerves will work in a dominant state when the pad of the thumb is placed on the palm side of the ring finger.

If you want immediate results, I think this form is effective.

I would like to introduce one more thing.

It's just a way to bend your ring finger just a little bit. Only this. This alone is surprisingly effective. It's a type that produces results slowly, even if it's not effective. It would be nice to incorporate it into the usual casual gestures.

Relax naturally.

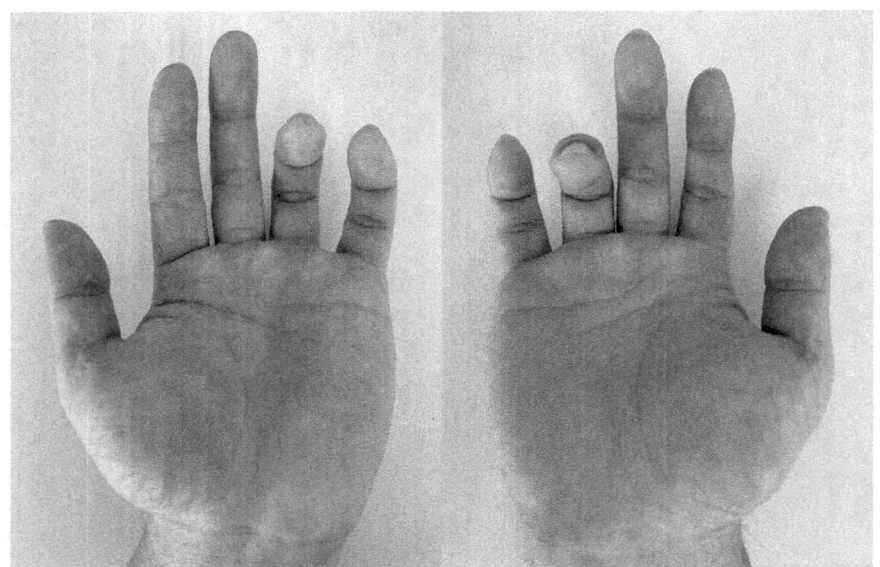

This is the secret of the ring finger. relaxation method. It's a way to unwind. Please try to remember when you are really in trouble.

Even so, the teaching continued. The story of Kagome, the story of Enma, and the revelation of a huge amount of information, I experienced the pain, anxiety, and fear that I didn't even feel like reading my notes because I was so scared. I don't feel like reading the memo.

Meaning of Enma

Beautiful to look at. Crown. Queen. The trajectory followed by those who are bestowed with the fruit of life. Enma is strangely scary when written in kanji, but its true meaning is Enma (a beautiful person who is extremely enthusiastic about one thing).

I would appreciate it if you could read it with the meaning of what I said.

Meaning of Kagome

Kagome, when written, it becomes the eyes of a basket. It means a picture pattern in which a triangle and an inverted triangle intersect. In simple terms, it is a diagram of light.

A close-up of a six-pointed star called Kagome.

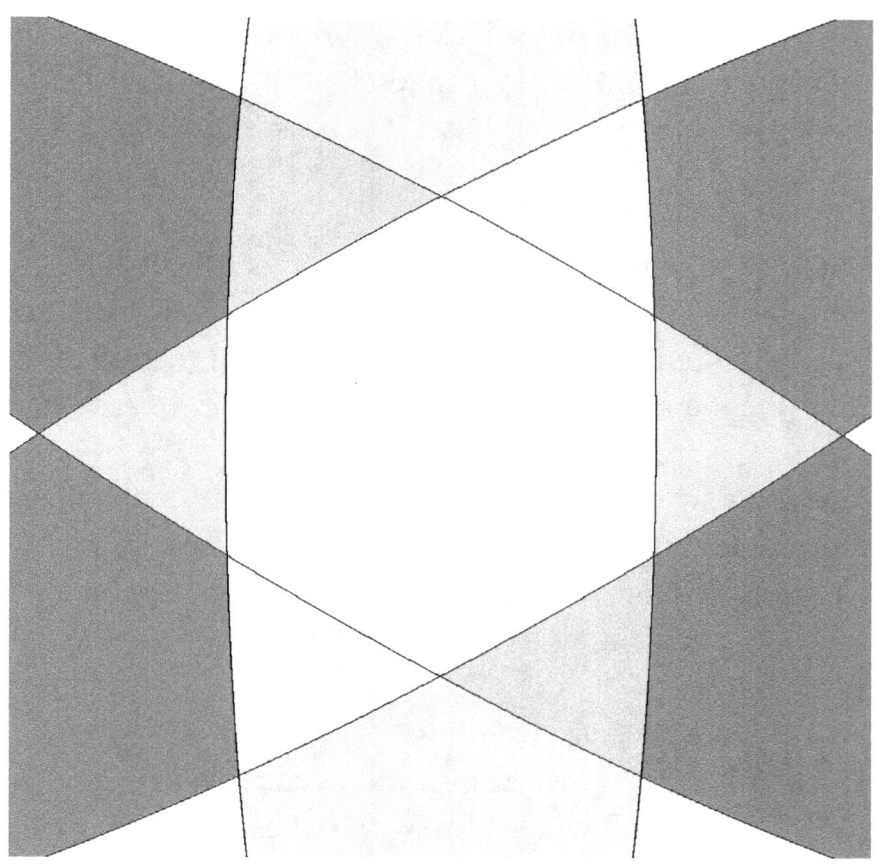

However, there is hope, and even in such a harsh situation, there is a real world that you can feel in the invisible world, and if you make a mistake, you will experience the pain of chills, fear and anxiety.

However, if you do it the right way, you can experience the feeling of bliss or paradise, where your heart and thoughts coexist. I am in a state of weakness. It is also a feeling of happiness and bliss. It was as if I was enjoying heavenly joy.

When I tasted that feeling, I thought, this is it, this is it. In order to taste this, I have continued the rising air current (ascension) every day. I feel like I'm recovering from the mental state that was bearish.

But here's where things become important. I don't know the reason, but as a result of continuing the ascending current, I will move to a state that can be said to be an ascending current (ascension) addiction.

When that happens, regardless of your will, the ascending current (ascension) will occur in quick succession, and it will be crazy regardless of the day or night. When this happened, I decided that I could not handle it by myself and started to rely on the hospital.

But be careful with this. The doctors are people who have never had an ascension experience. No matter how much you complain to the doctor about the current situation, they will only think of you as a crazy person. I pondered.

Ask yourself: Do you have the ability to explain the updraft (ascension) to others? My answer was NO. Therefore, even if you rely on the doctor, the answer will not be derived. There is no other way than to patiently interact with your own body and build a coping method.

However, in modern times, you can learn how to deal with it through books. Countermeasures are possible, and it gets a little better, and if you verify whether that method is correct or not, and if you make a distinction between what you should do and what you shouldn't do, you will gradually see the answer.

In my case, fortunately, I was blessed with books, and fortunately, I was able to verify my life pattern, thought pattern, and behavior pattern. Once I was able to do that, I was able to gradually reduce the anguish, chills, fear, and anxiety I had until then, and regained my composure.

And I have learned something. It seems that if only one side is raised, the judgment of Enma (crown, bean) will bring suffering, and chills, fears and anxieties will come to the surface and suffer.

I don't know why, but if I raise both sides instead of just one, it seems that I can enjoy the ultimate bliss and paradise.

However, when I evaluate it while admitting that I still need verification from now on, paradise and hell are two sides of the same coin, and depending on the person's thought pattern, behavior pattern, and life pattern, they can fall into either. I found out that.

I'll explain the thought pattern I'm getting right now. If you start chasing something you can't see, you should be the first to notice it and declare to yourself, "I will return to chasing something visible."

This allows you to escape from the fantasies and delusions associated with past memories. It also allows you to break away from the fantasies and delusions of the opposite non-existent future.

This is just a hypothesis, but I believe that we will be able to enjoy 100% paradise by enjoying bliss as it is, without imagining strange fantasies or delusions. Perhaps we are designed to experience suffering, chills, fear and anxiety when we cross that line.

For the time being, I've come to understand a little about that, so I'll report and explain.

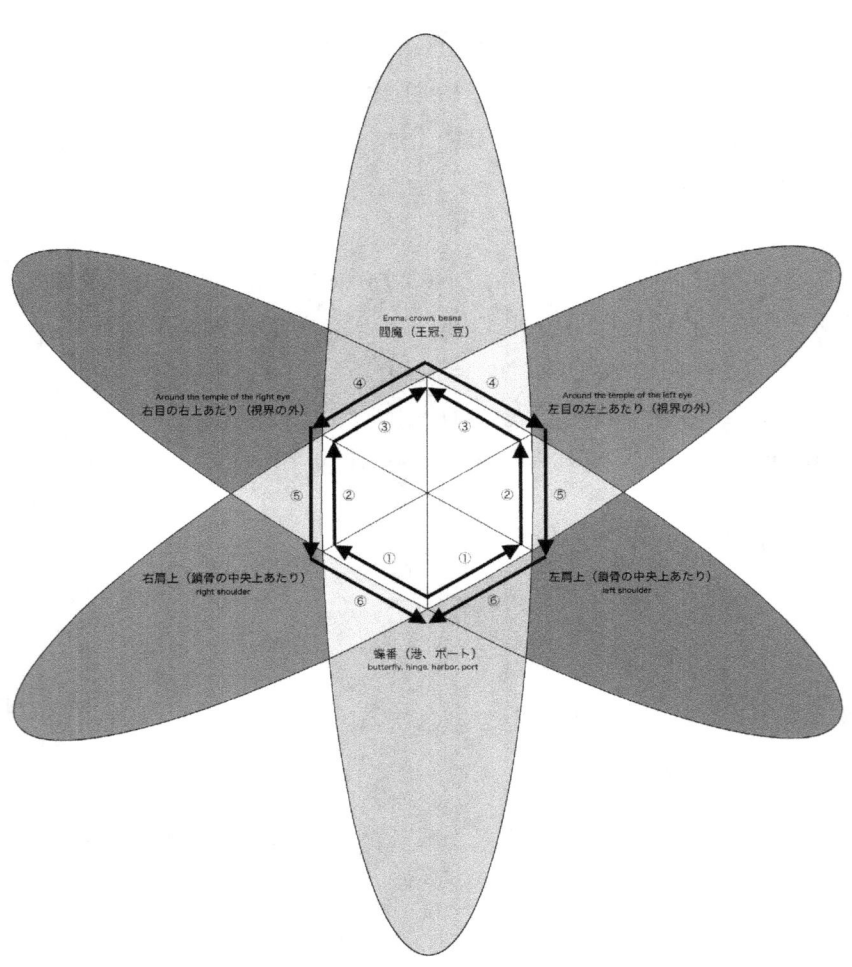

The hinge part (the part written as harbor or port) is the starting point. Then, follow the left and right routes at the same time and proceed to the destination called the Enma part (crown, bean) (1, 2, 3 in numerical notation are followed at the same time on the left and right).

This intentionally moves the heart energy up into the head energy. And when you reach the top, you wait for Enma's judgment. When Enma makes a decision, follow the left and right routes at the same time and return to the hinge part (harbor, port). (4, 5, and 6 in numerical notation are traced in order at the same time on the left and right)

This causes the energy of the head to intentionally descend into the energy of the heart. And you will come to taste the finest bliss and paradise. If you do not follow this method, it will turn into suffering (chills, fear, anxiety), so be careful.

Ah, yes, the hinge part (harbor, port). I will talk about where that position is based on my subjectivity. If you write it as it is, it may be taken like the center of the heart. I think we tend to think of it as the heart.

However, in my sense, it is a little higher position.

Since the feeling that I feel with my senses is like a butterfly, I express it as a hinge.

In terms of organs expressed in the world of medicine, I believe it is the thymus located above the heart.

You can't see it with your eyes. The fun is hidden there.

I thought that the crown might be associated with a wide circular part where the parietal bone and the parietal bone of the skull are sutured sagittal, so I dare to express it as a bean in order to express it with a dot.

Beans continue to rise (ascension) and appear at the end of their suffering. Words cannot explain it at all, so in medical terms, the suture between the frontal bone and the left and right parietal bones in the skull is called the coronal suture.

The point where the coronal suture and the sagittal suture intersect will be referred to as the position of the bean, or the position of Enma (crown, bean).

This is also similar to the thymus, and there is something interesting about it that cannot be seen with the naked eye.

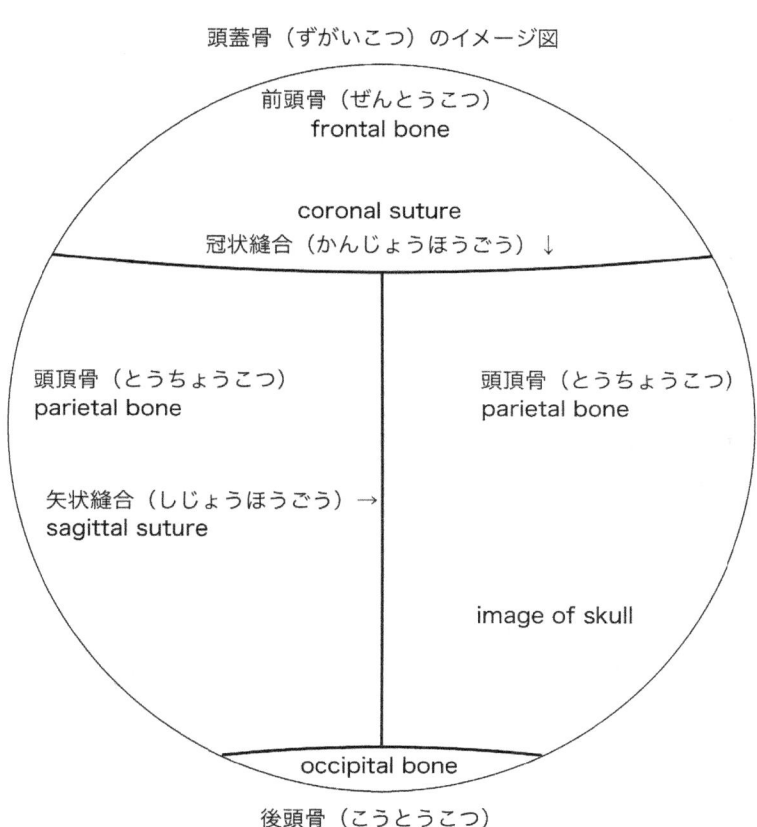

Also, the reason why it is called Enma is that the crown and the act of waiting for the bean's judgment is very similar to the image of Enma that appears in the Journey to the West and Dragon Ball, which I read long ago, so let me call it that.

The appearance of the life energy rising in a row from the hinge (thymus) in order reminds us of these stories, and is very similar. I thought.

Also, this name is a personal subjectivity, and I think it can be another name. Whether you call the top of your head the Last Judgment, or the center of your chest the Ark out of the harbor, I think you can call it anything.

The important thing is to raise the energy of the thymus (hinge, harbor, port) from both left and right, wait for the judgment of the top of the head (Enma, crown, bean), and after the judgment is given, let the energy go down to both the left and right. and return the energy to the thymus (hinge, harbor, port), which is also the hometown.

I think it's safe to call this Portland or Utopia. Also, I think that it will give glory to the world of later generations if we do not prescribe names.

Because I'm thinking about this, I'm in the shape of pursuing something invisible. Once I realize that, I will declare as I write this sentence, "I will return to chasing the visible world."

With this method, so far, I can enjoy the finest bliss and paradise without any problems. For the time being, I feel safe.

The reason I decided to publish this article is because I wanted to help people who are suffering from symptoms of ascension addiction.

Also, instead of expressing it as an ascending current, it is sometimes called the ascension of the Kundalini in the world of yoga. Therefore, it is my sincere hope that it can be a solution or a remedy for those who are in trouble with Kundalini syndrome.

Also, if you are interested in the updraft (ascension) on this occasion, I would like to give you one piece of advice. When preaching healing like this, there are cases where you are soliciting by claiming that you can get pleasure. Or you may be tempted by being touted as a way to get bliss.

But be careful. In exchange for that pleasure, the finest hell is also prepared. To be honest, I don't feel comfortable recommending the method of ascension to people because it can be a picture of life and death.

Based on my experience, I wouldn't recommend it.

If you follow a method that promotes the updraft (ascension), you will experience chills, fear, and anxiety, and will be invited to a life-and-death prospect. If you want to experience hell and get bliss, it's fine, but if you don't, it's better to never get involved.

Please take it as advice.

Also, if you still want to experience the ascending air current (ascension), we will clearly state that you are prepared to experience hell and that all responsibility lies with you.

In addition, we do not guarantee any damage to the customer's body after that. We ask that you proceed at your own discretion and at your own risk.

I, Mr. Takashi 2baki, will not be held responsible for any and all phenomena caused by the methods I introduce. Please note. Please do so at your own risk.

Please proceed only if you agree to this.

FOREWORD

*Caution: When the rising air current (ascension) begins to occur in the skull, it will be in a state of mental drowsiness (sleeping). You will not know if you are awake or asleep, and you will experience a state of meditation even if you do not meditate.

Also, if you have made a mistake in how to ascend, or if you are doing something that should not be done (thinking pattern, action pattern, life pattern, etc.), especially if it is your first experience, you may experience chills or You will be in a state of self-creating chills, fear, and anxiety.

It is possible that your body will become sensitive and sensitive, reacting to even trivial things, and that your mind and body will become easily out of balance. Special care must be taken in this situation.

MAIN STORY

From here, we will introduce how to heal to smoothly advance the ascending air current (ascension). We recommend that you proceed slowly without rushing. In fact, it will take many years for customers to reach the story of Enma. From my experience, it took 2 years and 10 months. Therefore, it is fine to think that it will take three years.

It will also take several months for the first updrafts (ascension) to occur. For me, it took 3 to 6 months. Therefore, I recommend that you keep going.

Also, there are three powers that are needed at this time. It is the imagination that willingly experiences the sensations of seeing, hearing, and feeling without resisting. The power of observation to observe what is happening in this body. Enthusiasm that can be called extraordinary enthusiasm to continue healing while enjoying it. With these three things, you'll definitely get there.

After the rising air current (ascension) begins to occur, I think that the phenomenon will make your heart flutter. It's going to be a really fresh and fun time, so please enjoy it to the fullest.

Now, let me teach you the basics of healing.

This time, I will introduce and give you the original text that I received the instruction.

CRYSTAL HEALING

A person who taught me crystal healing told me this.

Please choose the crystal (stone) that you are attracted to. Then I take a deep breath, close my eyes and bring the stone to my heart. Place both hands on your heart.

As you breathe in, please come to the inner being that resides within the stone. I will welcome you with a feeling of welcoming with my heart. As I exhale, I give the love and friendship that I have to the inner being that resides within this stone by saying, "Please take it."

Then, with each breath, exchange your current feelings. As you repeat it over and over, you will gradually feel that the energy is circulating, so continue to convey your feelings while breathing.

It is very important to offer love and gratitude to the stone. It is as important as welcoming the presence of the stone.

The reason why it is important is that this feeling of love and gratitude nourishes the stone. The stone receives nourishment. Feelings of love and gratitude are also very beneficial to the planet. It will nourish the earth.

If you interact with the stone with that feeling, the energy will gradually increase. Then, feedback from the other side is added each time, and it grows bigger each time.

And as it circulates and grows, it spirals out and forms one of the patterns for Ascension. Soon you will meditate with this stone being. And I will do it to meet and feel that existence.

Then, while breathing like before, convey your feelings, receive and give energy each time, and do it with your heart, gradually the presence of the stone will come into your heart. There are things that show you the image in your heart, so please experience it.

Then, when you see the image of the existence of the stone in your heart, ask a question. "What is your nature and what can I co-create with you?"

So, the response from the existence of the stone at that time may show us something. I may be able to show you something in the form of a reply from a stone being. They may send you images in the form of who they are. Or if you say "Please", the scenery will gradually change and you may be taken to various places on your journey.

And when an image, or a feeling of healing, comes to me, I don't resist, but gradually entrust it with the feeling of "Please show me more" and make it bigger and stronger. please And make a note of what happened.

Now close your eyes and get ready. Then focus on your breath and place the stone around your heart. Take a deep breath and start working.

End your meditation by thanking the stone beings. When you have finished thanking you, please slowly prepare and return here.

When you're done, it's a good idea to take notes before you forget. My book is made from this memo.

Is there anyone who has had a good feeling in their heart from this experience?

The good feeling that you are feeling in this heart is that feeling that your deep self, your deep self, is in motion.

And the next healing is especially important.

You will go through the process of encountering your deep self.

HOW TO MEET YOUR DEEP SELF

A person who taught me crystal healing told me this.

See the image of the cave opening into the heart. It will start descending from the mouth of the cave. Keep going down and down until you reach the bottom.

And when you get to the bottom, look around. I can see a faint light. If you look closely, you can see the door. You will see a door with your name on it. Knock on the door when you find it. Open the door and go inside.

someone is standing there. your inner deep self. Offer your love and friendship when you meet this being. And say thank you for opening the door at the bottom of your heart.

And question its existence. Ask, "What do you want me to tell you?" And for that matter, "What can I do?"

Whatever happens after that, let it happen without resistance.

And follow the way you came. Let's go back to the "heart". And take a break.

Now bring the stone to your heart and get ready for crystal healing. You go down from the heart into the cave, the downward cave, to meet the Deep Self in the depths of your heart.

Now let the crystal healing begin.

When you're done, clean up your mind and come back here.

Did you go down from the cave and meet your deep self? I believe this is the most important healing I can do. By doing this, you will allow your deep self to come to the surface and live with you.

You may feel that you and your deep self are actually one entity. When you get this complete picture, you will be able to live with your deep self in your daily life.

You need to merge and become one with your Deep Self. Most of the time, what happens is that when you connect with your Deep Self, you get your hands on it.

But sometimes you lose sight of it. and will come back. That kind of thing happens.

If you lose sight of your deep self, you can find it again by going into the cave and meeting again.

Next, I will introduce the healing that I usually do. This is a version of healing without the crystals. For the past two years, I have been doing this healing and causing an updraft (ascension).

USING LOVE AND FRIENDSHIP ENERGY

Place both hands on top of each other in the center of the heart.

Then, please exhale. When you have finished exhaling, inhale quickly and exhale slowly as you communicate to the existence within yourself.

I offer my love and friendship to you,
the being that is inherent in me.
I love you
I am friends with you.

Repeat this with each breath. If you have time now, let's meditate as it is. *Meditation time is free. I would like you to go as comfortable as you want.

Can any of you feel the energy of love and friendship emanating from the center of your heart? Or they may show us something in various forms, such as images, sounds, stories, etc.

If you feel that way, don't hold back and go ahead and experience it as if you want to see more. This is the proof that the existence inherent in the self is starting to move.

Also, make a note of what happens when you use the energy of love and friendship before you forget it.

My book is made from this memo.

This concludes the introduction to healing. As I introduced earlier, I had an ascension experience by continuing the crystal healing for about half a year. To describe the ascension in words, it can be said that the updraft has occurred at a level that can be felt in the body. And as a result of continuing it for 2 years and 10 months without getting tired of it, I was able to reach the phenomenon introduced at the beginning of this book. I would like to express my sincere gratitude to those who taught me crystal healing.

In addition, I would like to conclude the main part by introducing one breathing method as a countermeasure in the case that an ascending current (ascension) does not occur even after continuing this healing for half a year.

This breathing method is a strange experience that happened to me about 10 years ago when I was practicing a breathing method that I happened to read in a book when I didn't even know the word for ascending current (ascension).

This is the information that I think that it may be related to the rising air current (ascension) after that. It doesn't necessarily mean that you can't "ascend" without this breathing technique. I would like to offer and give it to those who have tried the healing described above for half a year and nothing happened.

BREATHING METHOD

Certainly, it was around 8 to 10 years ago from now when I was in my early 30s, so I don't remember exactly.

I was reading all sorts of yoga and self-help books, and there were several books that seemed to change your physical condition with your breath, and one of them had a breathing technique that focused on long exhalations. It was just a practice of exhaling long breaths earnestly.

If I remember correctly, the method was to open the mouth halfway, put the tongue on the upper jaw, exhale little by little, and gradually lengthen the exhalation time.

In the beginning, repeat exhaling for 4 seconds, then switch to 8 seconds when you can do it, and gradually increase the time, 10 seconds, 15 seconds, 30 seconds, and so on, and if I remember correctly, about 60 seconds. I was able to exhale for a long time, and when I was doing something challenging like how many times I could repeat it, suddenly, exhaling and inhaling occurred at the same time, and I was surprised and amused. I remembered that I was laughing.

I don't think I can do it now, but I remember being surprised at the time. I remember that at that time, I felt comfortable around the navel.

Thinking back on it now, I'm starting to think that maybe it played a part in the experience of the updraft (ascension) that would follow.

There is no particular scientific basis, but it is possible to provide information.

With that, I would like to conclude this volume. Thank you very much for reading. I pray from the bottom of my heart that a bright day will come to you. See you soon.

LITERATURE LIST

To become an obedient heart (Author) Konosuke Matsushita

Thinking about Humans (Author) Konosuke Matsushita

I asked a psychosomatic doctor who has zero recurrence rate after returning to work, "How to cure depression without relying on drugs" Satoshi Kamehiro (Author) Tatsuya Natsukawa (Author)

Martial arts fighter Katsunori Kikuno's who Tsuyo DOJOy
  https://www.youtube.com/watch?v=8H6LtISZ8Bw

Good sound is made with good posture and good breathing (Author) Shoji Mamada

Special Thanks : Robert Simmons

ABOUT THE AUTHOR

Born in Japan in 1981 AD and named Takashi 2baki. Upon graduating from high school, he moved to Tokyo to become an electrical engineer. He awakens to programming on the way, turns into a programmer and changes jobs to an IT company. At the timing when the Internet became completely popular, he moved to his hometown and changed jobs to a local company. While changing jobs repeatedly, he came into contact with the vision of doing what he likes as a job, and in view of the Internet business environment, which was rapidly developing, he made up his mind to become a self-produced musician. However, he didn't get the results he expected, and the trend changed, so he decided to turn his favorite natural stone into a business, and started a natural stone shop as Plan B. In the meantime, he got lucky and got an opportunity to meet the person who taught him crystal healing, and he was taught crystal healing directly. Since then, I have been working on writing.

Mr. Takashi 2baki

https://note.com/mr_takashi_2baki/

SERVICE

Even if you simply raise both, there are various ways to raise it. In my case, the way I ascend is changing day by day in accordance with the inner voice, the voice of the being that resides within me, the inner guidance, the sound of the bugs in my heart, or the spirit guide. With that in mind, it was good. I'd like to introduce you to the rising pattern that seems to be.

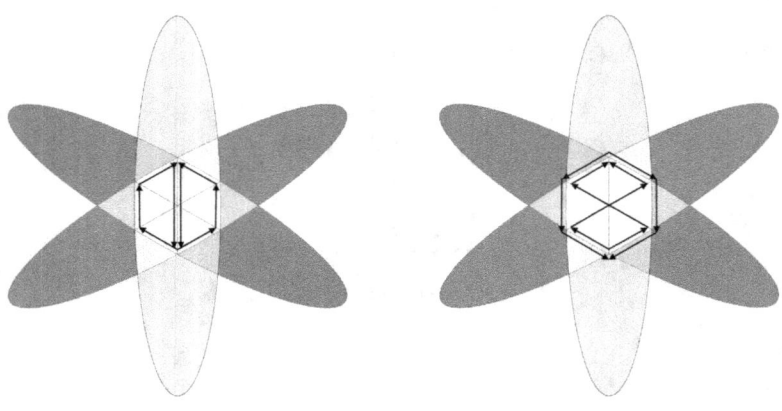

It also describes how the ascension was when good things happened.

I hope that it will be useful as a reference material.

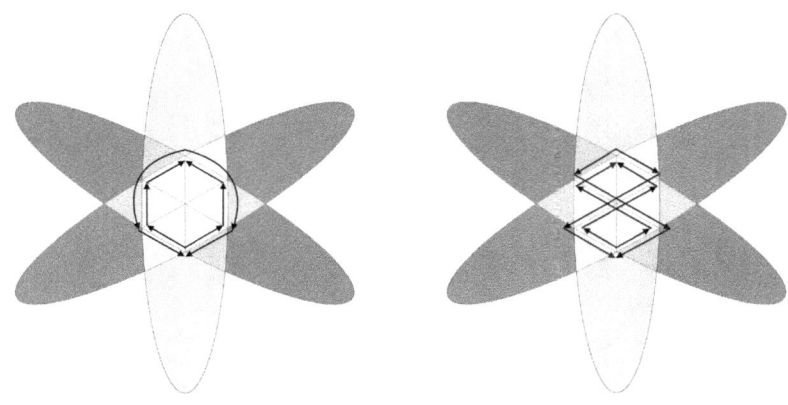

Painting by 2baki Takashi (1) [Energy Road]

I have put together a simplified image of what happened around mid-May 2022 during the transition to the awakening experience. The finer details will be kept confidential. The reason for keeping it secret is that details such as names and detailed orders may change the names and energy paths themselves depending on the person. The way it climbs will probably change, and the way it looks and perceives it will also change depending on the person. Also, if you specify or disclose your name, etc., the customer will be influenced by that name, and it may interfere with your own experience. In order to minimize the impact, detailed details such as names, designations, and nicknames will be kept confidential. It seems that something like this happened while being led to the awakening experience. I would appreciate it if you could see it to that extent.

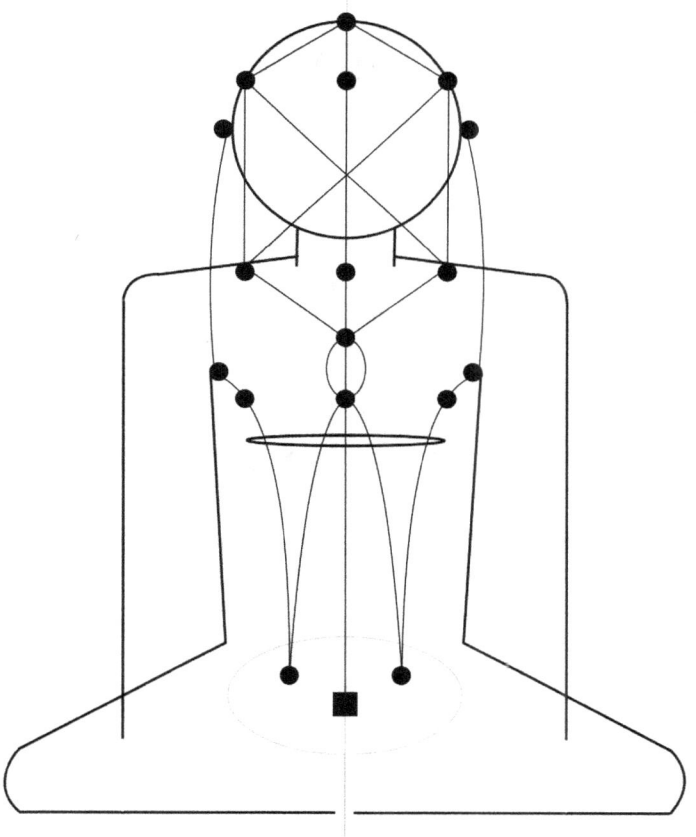

Painting by Takashi 2baki (2) [The Moon, the Sun and My Light]

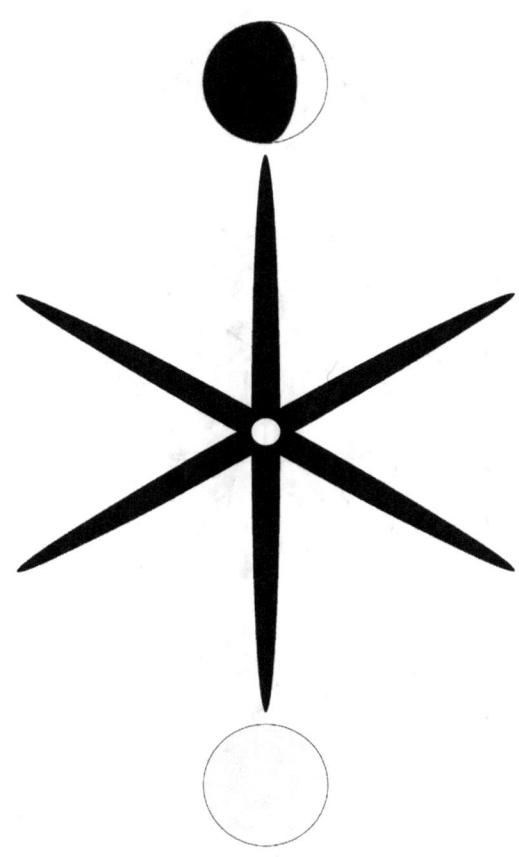

In the midst of hellish suffering, in the flow of rushing into the awakening experience, after the hexagram was clarified, there was a clarified word, and it is an image drawing based on that word. I hope you can enjoy the paintings without thinking about the deep meaning.

How to use the pendulum

This is what the person who taught me crystal healing said. I always ask my deep self how to use the pendulum and how to move it. Try asking something like, "Show me how it moves when you say YES," and observe how it moves in which direction. Then, ask the deep self, "Which direction and how is it 'NO' to move?" Then, I think that the difference between YES and NO will appear. And how it moves varies from person to person.

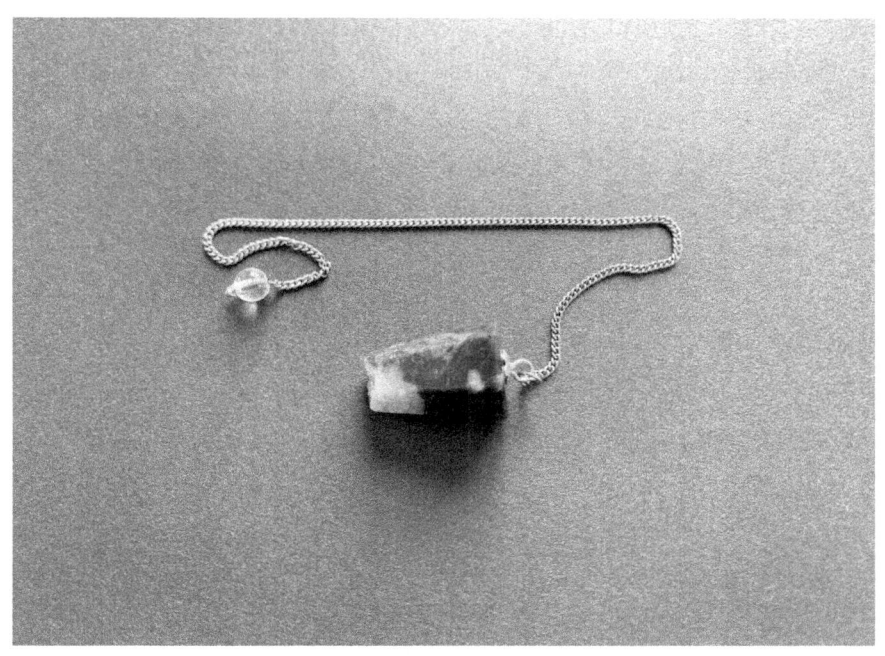

The three primary colors of light, the three primary colors of color, and the sign of light.

When I was studying visible light in quantum theory, I came to the three primary colors of light from the question that white and black do not exist. If you mix green, blue and red, you get white.

Also, black is called the three primary colors of color, and is a mixture of the three primary colors of light. Cyan is a mixture of green and blue, magenta is a mixture of blue and red, and yellow is a mixture of red and green. I learned that when these three colors are mixed, they become black.

The more I think about it, the more I wonder why. However, I think that colors are waves, and I wonder if black looks black because the waves cancel each other out and don't emit light. On the contrary, I wonder if white looks white because the waves are disturbed and emit light. That's how I interpret it.

sign of light

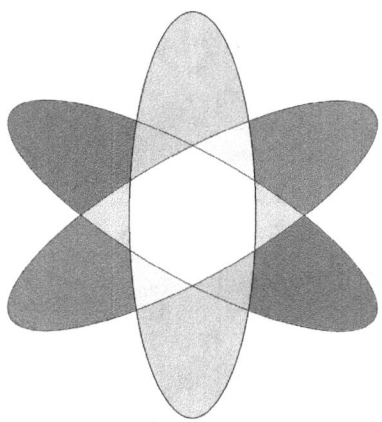

HYPOTHESIS

Thoughts after the Ascension Experience and the Awakening Experience

I hypothesize that everyone has an inner existence within themselves, and that they live their lives without being aware of this existence.

However, through inner inquiry, we are able to see with the mind's eye the presence within ourselves.

Only those who become aware of that existence can connect with it, communicate with it, receive its wisdom, enjoy its teachings, and know the fact that consciousness dwells in that existence.

And it is possible to share the identity of that existence (existence proof) like a dream. People have those qualities.

However, because the real world of the outside world passes by haphazardly, humans are well equipped to deal with it. As a result, I am considering whether I have forgotten the inner world.

I can't help but think that maybe this inner world was more natural in my childhood.

- However, in the process of becoming an adult, I forgot about this before I knew it. I believe that such a fact exists.

  However, humans who have noticed this experience an updraft (ascension) and are guided to an awakening experience.

  Knowing that this is the rule of this world, I write it down like a memorandum. good luck to you

This may be a matter of course, but a note

When talking to someone, look at their face when you speak.

If you talk without looking at the other person, for some reason it will not go well.

I wonder why…

Is it because if you don't ask the other person's complexion, you won't be in sync with the other person and the conversation will be one-sided? Or is it because, like the Internet space, the conversation becomes a string of characters, and it becomes an exchange in the brain space without facial expressions, like a conversation between thoughts…

I don't really know why, but

Anyway, it's better to talk while looking at the other person, so you can see the other person's signals, so the conversation progresses with the other person. There may be various reasons, but it is better to concentrate on the other person and talk while watching the situation of the other person.

It works better.

clash of ideas

Thoughts collide with each other, and if you move your head, they will collide. But think about what happens when you move with your mind.

Conclusion later…

Trigger your favorite meter.

It works only when the trigger of "I like this" works.

This is the first principle of action.

Other than that, I can't think of anything else.

No matter what.

Then love will be your guide.

Advice on self-love

Benefits of self-love.

Only when you can love yourself do you become spiritually independent.

Loving yourself means nourishing your body.

You will receive nourishment of love for your body.

There is nothing more reliable than this for my body.

A healthy feeling will grow, and a healthy feeling will be obtained. You can get those benefits.

Giving love and receiving love, such a cycle,

When the loop of love is born, this body will be in a joyful state and you will be happy from the bottom of your heart.

If you continue to do this, it will become a guidepost to your mental independence and will lead you to rise.

Yes, that's exactly why it will be your guidepost.

Thinking Criteria

When your thoughts are negative, you feel pain in your heart.

When your thoughts are positive, you feel comfort in your heart.

To give a more clear and easy-to-understand example, when you are in love. I think everyone has had the experience of thinking about someone they love so much that their hearts pounded and they couldn't stand still.

I think it's proof that something invisible exists in the center of the chest, the center of the heart.

Also, as you become aware of this, you will begin to turn your attention to the center of your heart. You will naturally observe the state of your heart. You will be able to instantly judge whether what you are thinking is good or bad, such as whether it is comfortable or not.

If you think it's comfortable, you can go ahead as it is, If you feel uncomfortable, stop thinking about it.

To put it another way, they serve as indicators for such judgment criteria.

I feel the possibility that the existence that becomes the core of that person is lurking in the center of the heart.

THYMUS

In the book I read at the library, there was information that I thought was this, so I'm going to quote it.

It's a medical book.

Even in neurophysiology, which has a short history and is difficult to establish an established theory, Dr. David Horobin of the Institute of Clinical Medicine in Montreal believes that a hormone called prostaglandin E1 is necessary for the smooth functioning of the immune system. claims that similar substances are very important.

Horobin, a scientist from Oxford University, also emphasizes that diet can modulate the immune system, especially T cells, which fight cancer.

Prostaglandin E1 is known to be abundantly stored in the thymus, where T cells mature.

If you create mice that lack T cells and have hyperactive B cells, they eventually die in a manner similar to mice with the autoimmune disease lupus erythematosus (SLE).

Horobin, however, discovered that when prostaglandin E1 was given to the mice, T cells returned to normal levels and B cell activity normalized, leading to longer life.

[Reference] Inner healing power New medicine concerning the mind and immunity (Authors) Stephen Locke + Douglas Corrigan (Supervision): Tojiro Ikemi (translation) Akira Tanaka + Masaaki Hori + Tetsuaki Inoue + Yasuko Urao + Keiichi Ueno

Even if you don't understand the meaning of the sentence, you can see that there is a place where a large amount of important "prostaglandin E1" is stored in the center of the chest, the thymus.

Shaking my head while reading, I thought, "Hmm." Also, at the end of the book, it says:

It's a fascinating therapeutic phenomenon that David McClelland has dubbed the "Mother Teresa Effect."

Mother Teresa is a Nobel Peace Prize laureate who dedicated her life to helping the poor of Calcutta. McClelland showed her students a moving film depicting her work, and was intrigued by the changes in her blood drawn before and after.

After watching the movie, the students' immunoglobulin levels rose slightly, suggesting that their immune systems functioned better.

Later, he confirmed this "Mother Teresa effect" in various ways. Instead of showing the film, he once asked graduate students to ponder two things.

In other words, it made me think about "when I was deeply loved by someone" and "when I loved someone" in my life. After all, it was effective.

In fact, McClelland had known about it experientially for a long time, and believed that it worked.

When I catch a cold, I think about the times when I loved and when I was loved. There have been two or three times when I've gotten over my cold just by doing that. That doesn't mean it will work for sure. No matter how much I tried, it didn't work, and there was a time when I had a bad cold. But it helps.

McClelland's strong belief in the power of love has great implications for the modern medicine he advocates.

This precious power of the human mind has hitherto been overlooked. But, according to him, that is the inner driving force in the phenomenon of therapy.

"By changing the hospital environment, we can do many things." McClelland once said at a meeting of medical professionals:

We need to make the hospital a place where people can relax, a place where compassion naturally arises, a place where they are freed from the constant feeling of being chased by something.

In other words, in a healthy environment. Doctors, nurses, and social workers can do it if they want to. Loving someone is very good for the health of the person you love. And, perhaps, you can expect an effect on the health of the loved one himself.

[Reference] Inner healing power New medicine concerning the mind and immunity
(Authors) Stephen Locke + Douglas Corrigan
(Supervision): Tojiro Ikemi (translation) Akira Tanaka + Masaaki Hori + Tetsuaki Inoue + Yasuko Urao + Keiichi Ueno

As I read this, I had the illusion that the use of love and friendship energy I was recommending was literally proven.

If we can confirm that the thymus is stimulated by practicing how to use the energy of love and friendship and strongly activates T cells, we can say that it is medically effective in suppressing cancer.

And, well, that's what I came up with. But I am neither a medical doctor nor a scientist, how can I confirm this? Right now, I haven't found an answer, so I'll put it on hold and move on.

T cells

In the thymus investigation, I was told that if T cells can be activated, the immune function can be improved and cancer can be suppressed. This time, we continued to investigate what T cells are. Even if I write it in my own words, it lacks persuasiveness, so I will quote the contents of the book.

The mechanism by which the immune system attacks cancer cells is gradually being understood.

One is by natural killer (NK) cells. NK cells have a primitive instinct, and as soon as they find something they are not, they attack and try to eliminate it. It has a very strong killing power, so there are many cases where cancers have shrunk dramatically by activating it.

NK cells are good at acting in a guerilla-like manner, rather than being systematically controlled.

Another is systematic immune activity centered on T cells (helper T cells, killer T cells, suppressor T cells).

Since T cells are governed by antigen-T cell receptor reactions that are very similar to antigen-antibody reactions, the process of recognizing antigens is necessary. Even if there are cancer cells nearby, T cells will miss them if they cannot recognize them as antigens.

Macrophages and dendritic cells called antigen-presenting cells inform T cells of the presence of antigens. Antigen-presenting cells ingest and digest cancer cells and pass on the information to helper T cells.

The helper T cells that receive the information release cytokines to make the killer T cells that attack cancer cells produce antigens and activate them to create a system to eliminate cancer cells.

[Reference] The definitive medical dictionary for cancer cures, from the latest modern medicine to reliable alternative therapies. Comprehensive dictionary for fighting cancer (General Supervisor) Ryoichi Obitsu

Shaking my head while reading, I thought, "Hmm."

I was impressed that humans have the ability to suppress cancer through a complex mechanism.

Even if you don't understand the content of the story, it would be nice if you could somehow understand that natural killer (NK) cells that move independently and T cells that move systematically are responsible for the body's immune function.

Of course, I have read and understood it, but I will write it with the meaning of a review.

To explain T cells that move systematically, killer T cells play a role in attacking cancer cells, and antigen-presenting cells (macrophages and dendritic cells) discover cancer. Then, it recognizes cancer, takes in cancer cells, conveys the information to helper T cells, and helper T cells release cytokines, present antigens to killer T cells, and activate killer T cells. T cells have a systematic mechanism to attack cancer cells after preparing to attack them.

As I read the book, I began to see how the cells in the human body work together to support the human immune system.

types of immune cells

I would like to organize the types of immune cells.

So far, I have written that T cells are active in immune function, but I have not mentioned what T cells are. I would like to break down that part here.

I imagine that there are many people who remember that human blood is made up of red blood cells, white blood cells, platelets, and plasma, a liquid component, that they learned in science or chemistry when they were students. This is the story of the white blood cells in it.

Leukocytes include lymphocytes, monocytes (macrophages, dendritic cells), and granulocytes. Lymphocytes in it include T lymphocytes, B lymphocytes, and natural killer (NK) cells. Among the T lymphocytes are killer T cells and helper T cells.

If you have read this far, you will notice that the T cells that we have explained so far are called T lymphocytes. If you can recognize that it is T lymphocytes (T cells) that come out of the thymus, you are in luck.

Helper T cells and cytokines

I will quote the description of cytokines produced by helper T cells.

Cytokines are proteins secreted from each cell, and as they are called intercellular communication molecules, carry various information and play the role of activating or calming cells according to the information.

We know that there are several types of cytokines, depending on their structure and action. Interleukins, interferons, and tumor necrosis factors are well-known cytokines related to cancer cells and immunity.

When cancer cells are found, macrophages and dendritic cells eat the cancer cells and their dead bodies, and at the same time, tell T cells what kind of cancer has developed. Upon receiving the information, the T cells are excited and activated. The helper T cells awaken the attacking force, the killer T cells, and attack the cancer cells.

Cytokines mediate this series of systems. IL-2, IL-12, etc. play a role in stimulus transmission. It is often said that immune cells are a very well-developed and elaborate system, but it is precisely because of cytokines that this system is able to function well.

[Reference] The definitive medical dictionary for cancer cures, from the latest modern medicine to reliable alternative therapies. Comprehensive dictionary for fighting cancer (General Supervisor) Ryoichi Obitsu

I will quote the description of helper T cells.

Advances in immunological research have revealed many interesting facts. One of them is that there are "humoral immunity" and "cellular immunity" in immunity.

"Humoral immunity" is immunity against fungi and bacteria. Macrophages and dendritic cells take up fungi and bacteria and pass on the information to helper T cells. There are two types of helper T cells, and type 2 helper T cells (Th2) are activated at this time. Th2 secretes IL-4, IL-5, IL-10, etc. to stimulate B cells and others.

Cell-mediated immunity is immunity against cancer cells. After engulfing cancer cells, macrophages and dendritic cells release IL-12, a cytokine that activates type 1 helper T cells (Th1). Th1 secretes IL-2 and interferon-γ (IFN-γ) to activate killer T cells and NK cells.

Humoral and cellular immunity are in a delicate balance with each other. It has been found that there is a relationship between the two cells, in which if one is too high, the other is suppressed.

In other words, in order for cell-mediated immunity, which attacks cancer cells, to work sufficiently, the action of humoral immunity must be suppressed.

Immunity has been described in terms of "increase" and "decrease" as a whole without distinguishing between "humoral" and "cellular". However, upon deeper study, it became clear that there is a delicate balance.

In order to treat cancer, it is meaningless unless cell-mediated immunity is enhanced.

For that purpose, it is necessary to promote the production of cytokines such as IL-12 and IFN-γ.

[Reference] The definitive medical dictionary for cancer cures, from the latest modern medicine to reliable alternative therapies. Comprehensive dictionary for fighting cancer (General Supervisor) Ryoichi Obitsu

Shaking my head while reading, I thought, "Hmm."

When you see technical terms, you tend to shy away from them before reading them, but what they are saying is simple. Our human body acquires humoral immunity against fungal and bacterial diseases by stimulating B cells via type 2 helper T cells.

In addition, against diseases caused by cancer cells and virus-infected cells (coronavirus and colds), cell-mediated immunity is acquired by activating killer T cells and NK cells via type 1 helper T cells.

These two immune functions work while maintaining a perfect balance, and if one increases, the other is suppressed.

What we can see from this is that T cells play a central role in controlling the immune system. I hope you can understand that this is the key point.

It is known that T cells are made from the thymus. If the thymus can be activated and a stable supply of T cells can be obtained, it will be possible to acquire well-balanced immunity against fungal and bacterial diseases, as well as cancer and virus-infected cell diseases (coronavirus and colds). We can assume that it will be possible.

We can see that cancer, corona, and most diseases depend on the work of T cells generated from the thymus. As long as you can activate the thymus, you can guess that there will be nothing to fear.

Autonomic nerves

We investigated the immune function centering on the autonomic nervous system. I will quote its contents.

Autonomic nerves are originally nerves that control the functions of the heart, gastrointestinal tract, respiratory system, blood vessels, and sweat glands. It is called the autonomic nervous system because it works independently without receiving commands from the brain. Even during sleep, when the brain is resting, the heart continues to work without rest due to the control of the autonomic nervous system.

The autonomic nervous system consists of the sympathetic and parasympathetic nervous systems, which have opposite functions. The sympathetic nervous system becomes dominant during exercise and tension, increasing the heartbeat, constricting blood vessels, and putting the body into an active state.

The parasympathetic nerves, on the other hand, are dominant at rest, slowing the heart rate and dilating blood vessels. By working the parasympathetic nerves, the mind and body are relaxed, and the secretion of digestive juices and defecation are urged.

White blood cells are one of the important components of blood along with red blood cells. Red blood cells carry nutrients and oxygen to cells and remove waste products and carbon dioxide.

On the other hand, white blood cells work to protect the body from infection and cancer. The ratio is 1 white blood cell to 1000 red blood cells.

Looking at the contents of white blood cells, in a healthy person, about 60% are granulocytes and about 40% are lymphocytes.

Granulocytes eat and process relatively large-sized foreign substances such as fungi, E. coli, dead cells, and molds. At this time, substances with strong oxidizing power (active oxygen) are released to destroy foreign substances. Active oxygen is greatly involved in the development and growth of cancer.

Lymphocytes are active in eliminating small foreign substances such as viruses. When lymphocytes recognize foreign substances as "antigens", they produce proteins called "antibodies" and work to detoxify the foreign substances. Types of lymphocytes include natural killer (NK) cells, T cells, and B cells.

There is a close relationship between autonomic nerves and white blood cells.

Autonomic nerves secrete neurotransmitters from nerve endings to regulate the function of internal organs. Adrenaline is released from the sympathetic nerves, and acetylcholine is released from the parasympathetic nerves, which give commands to the internal organs to induce tension and relaxation.

Adrenaline makes the mind and body tense. Increases heart rate and constricts blood vessels. Conversely, acetylcholine relaxes the mind and body. It also promotes digestion, absorption and excretion.

White blood cells, granulocytes and lymphocytes, respond differently to adrenaline and acetylcholine. Granulocytes are activated by adrenaline and inhibited by acetylcholine. Lymphocytes are the opposite.

In other words, when the sympathetic nerves become tense, adrenaline is secreted and granulocytes respond. When the parasympathetic nerve becomes dominant, acetylcholine is secreted and lymphocytes respond. To react means to activate and increase in number.

Granulocytes are cells that attack relatively large foreign substances that have invaded from the outside. It has an attack pattern that catches and melts, but it uses active oxygen as a weapon at this time.

Reactive oxygen is oxygen that is so unstable that it steals electrons from surrounding molecules in order to stabilize it. Molecules from which electrons have been deprived undergo a phenomenon called oxidation, and lose their activity all at once. It will rust and fall apart. Using this property, granulocytes process foreign substances.

When the sympathetic nervous system becomes tense and the number of granulocytes increases, the amount of active oxygen also increases.

Normally, active oxygen is removed by enzymes, but active oxygen generated beyond the ability of enzymes will attack regardless of the surroundings. Cells are oxidized and DNA is damaged. This leads to cell carcinogenesis. It also causes cancer cells to grow.

Active oxygen is also generated by respiration and cell metabolism. However, it is said that active oxygen emitted by granulocytes accounts for a considerable proportion. In other words, the more granulocytes there are, the more likely cancer is to develop.

For cancer treatment, it is better not to increase granulocytes. An increase in granulocytes means a relative decrease in lymphocytes.

As granulocytes increase, cells become cancerous due to active oxygen, and as lymphocytes, which eliminate cancer cells, decrease, immunity weakens. Therefore, it can be said that it is the best environment for cancer cells to live.

In other words, in order to cure cancer, it is necessary to reduce the number of granulocytes that generate active oxygen and increase the number of lymphocytes that try to eliminate cancer, thereby creating an environment in which cancer cells cannot survive.

Factors that cause cancer.

· Overworked and lack of sleep

It is good if you are getting enough sleep, but if you are working continuously with 3 to 4 hours of sleep, the number of granulocytes will increase abnormally, the amount of active oxygen will increase, and the cells will be oxidized.

· Trouble of heart

Stress such as anxiety, worry, and sadness is sensed in the brain's limbic system and transmitted to the hypothalamus.

The hypothalamus is a place that controls the autonomic nervous system and endocrine. When the hypothalamus receives a stress stimulus, it secretes adrenaline and noradrenaline, creating a state of sympathetic nervous tension.

As a result, your heart rate and breathing speed up, and your blood pressure rises. We all know that anxiety makes your heart beat faster.

By increasing the number of granulocytes, decreasing the number of lymphocytes, and impairing blood flow, it creates an environment for cancer to develop and proliferate.

In order to suppress the growth of cancer cells and bring them to treatment, it is necessary to increase lymphocytes and boost immunity.

Lymphocytes can be increased by making the parasympathetic nerves dominant.

[Reference] The definitive medical dictionary for cancer cures, from the latest modern medicine to reliable alternative therapies. Comprehensive dictionary for fighting cancer (General Supervisor) Ryoichi Obitsu

What is a granulocyte?

It is a general term for white blood cells that have "granules" containing components with bactericidal action in the cells. They are divided into three types: neutrophils, eosinophils, and basophils.

[Reference] Homepage of the National Cancer Center

Shaking my head while reading, I thought, "Hmm."

I thought it would be nice to think that the sympathetic nerves and parasympathetic nerves work together while balancing each other, just like two types of helper T cells.

Perhaps both are necessary, and I interpret that we are required to live in a balanced manner. I think that if you try to sleep with the sympathetic nervous system dominant during the day and sleep with the parasympathetic nervous system dominant at night, you will have a well-balanced life cycle.

Finally, I found it. How can I show that my immunity has increased? In other words, what is the object of evaluation that can be judged? How can I get the numerical data? I found the criteria for that.

Evaluation criteria for autonomic nervous system immunotherapy.

Treatment is carried out while confirming the effect by checking the number of lymphocytes and the percentage of white blood cells.

In the case of a healthy person, 1 mm^3 (cubic millimeter) of blood contains about 2300 to 2600 lymphocytes.

About 2,000 is the lower limit, and it is said that if the number is less than this, the immune system will be weakened and people will become more susceptible to illness.

For cancer patients, 1500 is quite good. 1500 or less. It is said that there are cases where it is about 1000, or even less, when receiving treatment such as anticancer drugs.

The goal of autonomic nervous system immunotherapy is to restore the number of lymphocytes to about 2000. When it exceeds 2000, the immune force gradually gains strength.

[Reference] The definitive medical dictionary for cancer cures, from the latest modern medicine to reliable alternative therapies. Comprehensive dictionary for fighting cancer (General Supervisor) Ryoichi Obitsu

I wanted this. This. what i wanted to find out.

I realized that I should evaluate how to use the energy of love and friendship based on this.

If you are reading this and have a cancer patient close to you, Teach them how to use the energy of love and friendship as soon as possible. Worth a try.

From now on, I would like to proceed with my own research.

However, it is not something that can produce results right away.

This is because it is not medically recognized unless it clears what is called a clinical trial.

Therefore, it is not something that can be achieved overnight.

Summary of Thymus

Is there a medical basis for using the energy of love and friendship? I will answer that question. There is a fact that some medical scientists are expecting the effect of the power of love on the immune system. There is a fact that the thymus, the main organ that controls human immune function, is hidden in the heart. We conclude that there is room for further research.

Also, there is an open issue. At present, there is no evidence that using the energy of love and friendship can medically stimulate the thymus gland, affect T cells that control immune function, and improve human immune function.

As a future task, I think that we will be able to see how much the immune function will be affected by collecting blood before and after using the energy of love and friendship, and how much effect will be obtained. In addition, you will be evaluated by looking at the results of using the energy of love and friendship continuously for 6 months to 3 years. If we can investigate how much influence appears and how much effect can be obtained, I hope that it will be proven as a method of improving immunity medically.

If the expected results can be obtained, it is speculated that there is a hidden possibility that it can be used in cancer treatment in combination with existing treatment methods.

If it is proved that there is medical evidence and scientific evidence on how to use the energy of love and friendship, it will be possible to reduce the anxiety of people living in Fukushima Prefecture who are afraid of cancer. I hope it will be possible.

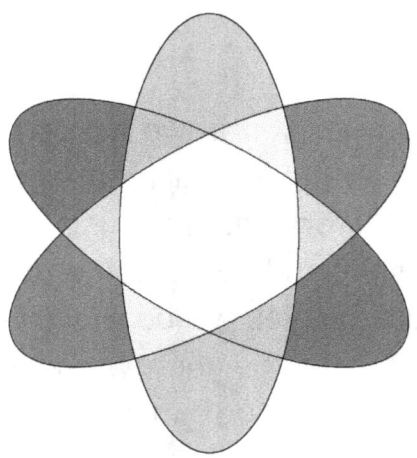

A story about experiencing the activation of the thymus

There are things I think about after experiencing an ascending current (ascension) experience and an awakening experience.

One of the phenomena that occurs around the climax of ascension is the activation of the thymus. Activation of the thymus occurs at a level that can be felt through the skin.

If I were to put the phenomenon at that time into words, I would say that I felt an energy body in the center of my heart, a little above my heart, like a hinge like a butterfly. You might call it wings. It may not be an exaggeration to describe it as a bird of a burning hot sun.

When I felt the sensation of the thymus, I was associated with the word "small 4". I remember the feeling I had when I was in 4th grade, and I think that feeling back then was the most correct. And I think it's the best. I remembered. It feels like when the gender distinction wasn't so big... when everyone was friends.

It seems that the time when the thymus is most activated in one's lifetime peaks around the fourth grade of elementary school. It is said that the thymus will continue to atrophy for the rest of one's life, with a peak in the 4th grade of elementary school, until the age of 70. I was surprised that it matched the experience associated with "4th grade". If you convert "4th grade" into age, it is 10 years old.

[Reference] Wikipedia research https://ja.wikipedia.org/wiki/%E8%83%B8%E8%85%BA

Come to think of it, the difference between men and women began to appear after that time, and before I knew it, there was a big difference between me physically and mentally.

I remember that something like that happened a long time ago.

I remember that even if I got injured at that time, it healed well. I realized again that the healing power at that time was thanks to the thymus.

In addition, when the thymus is activated by the ascending air current (ascension) experience and the awakening experience, you can feel as if you have regained the mind of a child.

It's a feeling that you can really taste the feeling of childhood.

You can say it's an innocent heart, or you can say it's a sense of enjoying everything, it's a very good and rich feeling that you're always happy and enjoying yourself and always smiling.

If you are dissatisfied with modern society and have a sense of being unrewarded or unsaved, why don't you experience this feeling once?

When you come to be able to enjoy that feeling, your perspective and way of thinking will be renewed, and you will be able to live with satisfaction. I would appreciate it if you could convert it to such a life.

Blood test results. facts on the surface, facts on the back

For a moment of joy, I will pick up the numbers that have been seen in the blood test. Historical blood test data.

採取日付 採取時間 伝票名	2016/05/10	2022/02/16 検体検査	2022/03/09 検体検査	2022/05/18 検体検査
WBC	6120	5240	5450	6780
RBC	563	550	565	552
Hgb	16.0	16.3	16.6	15.5
Hct	47.0	49.0	49.7	46.8
MCV	83	89	88	85
MCH	28.4	29.6	29.4	28.1 L
MCHC	34.0	33.3	33.4	33.1
PLT	24.9	31.9	34.7	37.9
白血球像				
Baso	0.3	0.6	0.7	0.6
Eosino	7.7 H	4.4	8.4 H	3.4
Stab				
Seg				
Neutro	62.3	53.4	46.0	62.7
Lympho	18.8	35.7	39.6	26.7
Mono	10.9 H	5.9	5.3	6.6
その他1	0.0	0.0	0.0	0.0
その他2	0.0	0.0	0.0	0.0
EBL		0.0	0.0	0.0
リンパ球（実数）	1150.0 L	1870.0 L	2160.0	1810.0 L
好中球（実数）	3810.0	2800.0	2500.0	4250.0
LD/IFCC		148	142	153
CK	83	436 H	90	166
BUN	15.3	11.6	11.9	18.0
CRE	0.91	0.93	0.91	0.84
UA		6.7	5.8	6.0
Na	142	142	142	142
K	3.9	3.9	3.7	3.7
Cl	102	106	105	104
HDL-C		43	40	38 L
LDL-C		172 H	195 H	197 H

February 16, 2022 is the day when I was asked to undergo a medical checkup again for the first time and received it at my family hospital. On this day, he underwent an echocardiogram of the heart and was diagnosed as having no abnormalities. At this time, I was told that my LDL-C, so-called LDL cholesterol, was high and that I should try to lower it.

March 9, 2022, this day is the 1th transitional observation day. You can see the numbers getting worse. At that time, I thought it would be okay because I stopped drinking drinks, which had been my daily routine, for a month. However, the results are coming out, and I'm going to be urged to change my mindset. Then, with advice from a dietician, I developed a habit of moderate exercise (walking) and adopted diet therapy.

May 18, 2022, this day is the second transitional observation day. Personally, I was confident, but the results were even worse, why? Why? It was a result that I thought even though I did that much. However, blood test results were worse, but there was a fact that the weight was drastically reduced. The doctor in charge told me to observe the progress without prescribing medicine because I could see the traces of my efforts. And the day ended with the story that I will see the doctor again in 3 months.

I also got advice from a nutritionist. This is a cooking method to make "Instant noodles in a bag". Until then, the soup, ingredients (cabbage, etc.) and noodles were boiled together and eaten as is. However, the proposed method was to boil the noodles and soup separately, and then drain the noodles. Then, he taught me a cooking method that turns that rich ramen into a light ramen, and I remember suddenly being motivated to do it.

Also, I changed my walking method from walking around the baseball field in the sports park to walking while observing the scenery. For example, I made a route to walk to the library, cool down at the library, read while I was in the mood, resume walking when I felt better, and go home.

Walking in circles around the same place is boring because it has no purpose, but I realized that walking with a motivation to read a book can be surprisingly enjoyable.

Among them, I gave myself various rewards, such as drinking pineapple juice when I could walk halfway, and devised ways to do it.

August 10, 2022

And then, on August 10, 2022, the long-awaited day came. I got results. If you observe the place where LDL cholesterol is written, you will see that the value of LDL cholesterol is decreasing.

No	検査項目	結果	下限値	上限値	コメント	コメント2	単位名称
1	白血球数	5590	3500	9700			/MCL
2	赤血球数	533	M438	577			マン/MCL
3	血色素量	15.0	M13.6	18.3			G/DL
4	ヘマトクリット	46.2	M40.4	51.9			%
5	MCV	87	M 83	101			FL
6	MCH	28.1 L	M28.2	34.7			PG
7	MCHC	32.5	M31.8	36.4			%
8	血小板数	29.9	14.0	37.9			マン/MCL
9	白血球像						
10	好塩基球	0.5	0.0	2.0			%
11	好酸球	5.0	0.0	7.0			%
12	桿状核球		0.0	19.0			%
13	分葉核球		27.0	72.0			%
14	好中球	45.2	42.0	74.0			%
15	リンパ球	42.9	18.0	50.0			%
16	単 球	6.4	1.0	8.0			%
17	その他1	0.0		0.0			%
18	その他2	0.0		0.0			%
19	赤芽球	0.0		0.0			/100WBC
20	リンパ球（実数）	2400.0		GT 2000			/MCL
21	好中球（実数）	2520.0					/MCL
22	LD/IFCC	136	120	245			U/L
23	CK	109	M 50	230			U/L
24	尿素窒素	14.6	8.0	20.0			MG/DL
25	クレアチニン	0.93	M 0.65	1.09			MG/DL
26	尿酸	6.7	M 3.6	7.0			MG/DL
27	ナトリウム	142	135	145			MEQ/L
28	カリウム	4.1	3.5	5.0			MEQ/L
29	クロール	108	98	108			MEQ/L
30	総コレステロール	212	150	219			MG/DL
31	中性脂肪	206 H	50	149			MG/DL
32	HDLコレステロール	40	M 40	80			MG/DL
33	LDLコレステロール	155 H	70	139			MG/DL

However, there is a caveat. I was advised by a nutritionist. What kind of drink do you drink when you walk? I was asked, so I immediately answered that it was pineapple juice. Then, the nutritionist seemed to get the point and said "That's it". I was so surprised that my eyes popped out. smile.

Apparently, when you drink sweet drinks, it seems that " neutral fat " will be high. Therefore, when walking, it would be difficult to completely quit pineapple juice, so he told me to alternate drinking with green tea or barley tea.

With that said, I will leave the visible story to this point, and from here on I will talk about things that blow away common sense. It's an invisible story.

From July 10, 2019, I was taught crystal healing, and as a result of performing it almost every day, I experienced ascension half a year later. Since then, I have spent my days ascending almost every day, and around mid-May 2022, I had an awakening experience accompanied by a frightening experience. In the process of moving to the awakening experience, I happened to have a blood test.

Let's take a look at the materials for May 18, 2022.

Blood test results on May 18, 2022

No	検査項目	結果	下限値	上限値	コメント	コメント2	単位名称
1	白血球数	6780	3500	9700			/MCL
2	赤血球数	552	M438	577			マン/MCL
3	血色素量	15.5	M13.6	18.3			G/DL
4	ヘマトクリット	46.8	M40.4	51.9			%
5	MCV	85	M 83	101			FL
6	MCH	28.1 L	M28.2	34.7			PG
7	MCHC	33.1	M31.8	36.4			%
8	血小板数	37.9	14.0	37.9			マン/MCL
9	白血球像						
10	好塩基球	0.6	0.0	2.0			%
11	好酸球	3.4	0.0	7.0			%
12	桿状核球		0.0	19.0			%
13	分葉核球		27.0	72.0			%
14	好中球	62.7	42.0	74.0			%
15	リンパ球	26.7	18.0	50.0			%
16	単　球	6.6	1.0	8.0			%
17	その他1	0.0		0.0			%
18	その他2	0.0		0.0			%
19	赤芽球	0.0		0.0			/100WBC
20	リンパ球（実数）	1810.0 L		GT 2000			/MCL
21	好中球（実数）	4250.0					/MCL
22	LD/IFCC	153	120	245			U/L
23	CK	166	M 50	230			U/L
24	尿素窒素	18.0	8.0	20.0			MG/DL
25	クレアチニン	0.84	M 0.65	1.09			MG/DL
26	尿酸	6.0	M 3.6	7.0			MG/DL
27	ナトリウム	142	135	145			MEQ/L
28	カリウム	3.7	3.5	5.0			MEQ/L
29	クロール	104	98	108			MEQ/L
30	総コレステロール	241 H	150	219			MG/DL
31	中性脂肪	125	50	149			MG/DL
32	HDLコレステロール	38 L	M 40	80			MG/DL
33	LDLコレステロール	197 H	70	139			MG/DL

At this time, I have not yet had an awakening experience. However, there is no doubt that it was a process of transitioning to an awakening experience. I recall that I was in the midst of a so-called fearful experience. To be precise, on May 27, 2022, I am stuck at the hospital. Around May 21, 2022, there is evidence that a closing coupon was issued that decided to close the natural stone shop that was selling online at that time, so it was probably around the time when Kagome's story appeared.

I can only say that it is a miracle that there is a blood document from that time. I think I had a blood test at a good timing. And now I am grateful for the health checkup.

In fact, when asked when I had my awakening experience, I honestly don't know when I had my awakening experience. I think it was around the beginning of June 2022.

The reason why this precious experience has become ambiguous is that in the process of moving on to the awakening experience, I was really in the process of letting go of everything. He also closed the Tennen Ishiya, which he had started at a cost of 2 million yen, discontinued all the books he had published up to that point, and completely deleted the accounts he had posted up to that point. And, well, well, there are no records left.

In fact, at the time, I couldn't do anything.

Because I was reluctant to even tell people about healing. If healing causes such pain, it would be better not to teach it. In the first place, it is not necessarily the case that there are people who want ascension and awakening experiences. I was thinking that if it was just my self-satisfaction, I should stop telling them.

However, after that experience, my body returned to normal, my mind became healthy, and I made an unexpected discovery. A thymic sensation that occurs in the process of transitioning to an awakening experience. When I started to think that maybe someone in the world could be saved if I taught healing using this thymus sense, it became the driving force to teach healing.

The thymus plays a central role in human immune function, and it is now known that it is an organ that matures T cells (T lymphocytes) that protect the body from corona and cancer. Even though I am an amateur, I can't help thinking that if we can activate the thymus, we can say that we can strengthen and improve the human immune function.

It was only after I realized this that I was able to open the Thymus Activation Healing to the public.

Also, on July 19, 2022, there was a corona-positive patient at home, and I was quarantined for about a week according to the instructions of the public health center.

At that time, I did thymus activation healing and saw what would happen. When I tried it, I myself had symptoms that made my throat irritated, but I didn't have any symptoms such as coughing or fever, and I was able to spend a week of quarantine safely.

I don't know if it just happened that I didn't get the coronavirus or because of the thymus activation healing, but I was able to escape the difficulty.

In addition, when I taught the thymus activation healing to the corona-positive patients and observed their progress, they did not become severe. Of course, I think it was because of the medicine, but I have received reports from corona-positive patients that they felt better after performing thymus activation healing.

By the way, my family is all rare unvaccinated people. Even in such an environment, there are no serious corona patients.

After this experience, I went to the hospital on August 10, 2022 and received a blood test.

If you compare the results of a blood test miraculously performed in the process of moving to the Awakening Experience and the results of a blood test after overcoming the corona after going through the Awakening Experience, you will see interesting results.

May 18, 2022 (Before Awakening Experience)
Lymphocyte count (real number) 1810.0/MCL
Neutrophils (real number) 4250.0/MCL

August 10, 2022 (after the awakening experience)
Lymphocyte count (real number) 2400.0/MCL
Neutrophils (real number) 2520.0/MCL

Of course, considering that pollen and mold grow in May, there will be seasonal changes in the numbers. It does not necessarily mean that it is good if the lymphocyte count is rising, but it is required that it is in balance.

This is because when the lymphocyte count is abnormally high, it is suspected as a disease, and when the lymphocyte count is abnormally low, it is suspected as a disease.

Therefore, it is not necessarily the case that the larger the quantity, the better. The key is to be balanced, yet activated.

Therefore, I am aware that it is not possible to judge that the thymus is activated from this value. I think the numbers are good as a result. I'm healthy now.

Also, I am aware of the current situation that no method has been found to evaluate that the thymus has been activated by thymus activation healing. I would like to know how to evaluate that the thymus is activated.

I can see the answer, but how to prove it is a mystery.

I am convinced that this will be an issue for the future.

AT THE END

If you practice how to use energy using love and friendship in the main story, after about 3 to 6 months, an ascending current (ascension) will occur that will become a dragon rising to your heart.

When the first ascension occurred, I was amazed. You will come to realize how wonderful it is to use the energy of love and friendship.

I came to believe that the ascension was a real thing, a real story.

And as a result of continuing the ascending current, the ascending current moves from the heart to the back of the throat.

Furthermore, as you continue to advance the updraft (ascension), you will move into the skull. But so far, it's pure pleasure. It felt good and I was happy.

However, in my example, after two years and ten months of practicing the use of love and friendship energies, the ascension moved into the skull and then into the crown of the head. In the midst of the shifting updraft, hellish torments emerged.

It's completely different from the pleasure until then, and I'm going to suffer. I was tormented by chills, fear and anxiety. Then it evolved into an updraft (Ascension) of shared suffering and joy.

The ensuing awakening experience is described in detail in this book. Please loop this book and read it.

Finally, I will teach you about thymus activation healing.

Thymus Activation Healing

I would like to tell you in your youth.

First, place your left thumb on your left clavicle and your left index finger on your right clavicle. Place your right thumb above your left index finger and your right index finger above your left thumb.

It's not accurate, but imagine that the thymus is roughly around that area. In the first place, the position of the thymus is to be experienced in the process of advancing to the awakening experience, so I will avoid mentioning it here.

Focus your attention on your breathing.
Say it with your heart as you exhale.

"I dedicate my love and friendship to you."
"I love you."
"I'm friends with you."

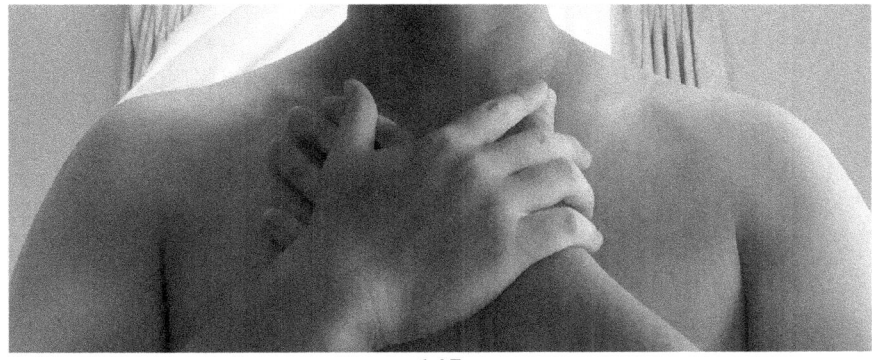

Don't say it out loud, but mutter in your heart. Repeat with each breath. If you have time now, let's just meditate. *There is no set time to meditate. I would like you to go as comfortable as you want.

Can anyone feel the energy of love and friendship emanating from the center of their hearts?
Alternatively, they may show us something in various forms, such as images and visions, sounds and music, videos and stories.

If you feel that way, don't hold back and go ahead and experience it as if you want to see more of it. This is the proof that the existence inherent in the self is starting to move.

Also, before you forget what happened when you used the energy of love and friendship, make a note of it.

My book is made from this memo.

www.ingramcontent.com/pod-product-compliance
Lightning Source LLC
Chambersburg PA
CBHW050003230526
45465CB00003BB/1240